Chinese National Health Care Reform

Five years have elapsed since the Chinese government announced its ambitious health care reform programme. The fact that both the United States and China unfolded their gigantic national health care reforms almost simultaneously is reflective of the daunting health policy challenges that most national governments are grappling with. While Obamacare has barely survived the obstruction from Congress and remains controversial, its Chinese counterpart has concluded its first phase at a fairly smooth pace. Having had three trillion RMB invested into it within five years, this landmark reform stands out as one of the biggest health policy interventions in modern history in terms of both scale and scope. A critical juncture in the reform process has been reached and it is time to assess its performance to date. This book provides an interim evaluation of China's ongoing national health care reform from an interdisciplinary perspective. Insights generated are not only valuable to inform the next phase of the reform, but also relevant to health policy reformers in other developing and transitional countries.

This book was published as a special issue of the *Journal of Asian Public Policy*.

Alex Jingwei He is the Associate Head of the Department of Asian and Policy Studies at the Hong Kong Institute of Education. He co-edits the *Journal of Asian Public Policy*. He specializes in health policy and reforms with particular reference to East Asia.

Qingyue Meng is a leading expert in health policy and economics. He has widely published in many prestigious journals. He is the Dean of the School of Public Health at Peking University, Beijing, China, and a key health policy advisor to the Chinese government.

Chinese National Health Care Reform

On the mend?

Edited by
Alex Jingwei He and Qingyue Meng

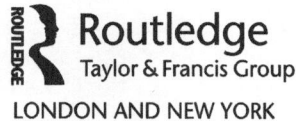

LONDON AND NEW YORK

First published 2016
by Routledge
2 Park Square, Milton Park, Abingdon, Oxon, OX14 4RN, UK

and by Routledge
711 Third Avenue, New York, NY 10017, USA

First issued in paperback 2017

Routledge is an imprint of the Taylor & Francis Group, an informa business

British Library Cataloguing in Publication Data
A catalogue record for this book is available from the British Library

ISBN 13: 978-1-138-09909-8 (pbk)
ISBN 13: 978-1-138-93678-2 (hbk)

Typeset in Times New Roman
by RefineCatch Limited, Bungay, Suffolk

Publisher's Note
The publisher accepts responsibility for any inconsistencies that may have
arisen during the conversion of this book from journal articles to book chapters,
namely the possible inclusion of journal terminology.

Disclaimer
Every effort has been made to contact copyright holders for their permission to
reprint material in this book. The publishers would be grateful to hear from any
copyright holder who is not here acknowledged and will undertake to rectify
any errors or omissions in future editions of this book.

Contents

Citation Information

The chapters in this book were originally published in the *Journal of Asian Public Policy*, volume 8, issue 1 (March 2015). When citing this material, please use the original page numbering for each article, as follows:

Chapter 7

The impact of China's Zero-Markup Drug Policy on county hospital revenue and government subsidy levels
Zhongliang Zhou, Yanfang Su, Benjamin Campbell, Zhiying Zhou, Jianmin Gao, Qiang Yu, Jiuhao Chen and Yishan Pan
Journal of Asian Public Policy, volume 8, issue 1 (March 2015) pp. 102–116

For any permission-related enquiries please visit:
http://www.tandfonline.com/page/help/permissions

Notes on Contributors

Benjamin Campbell is based in the Department of Anthropology at Dartmouth College, Hanover, New Hampshire, USA.

Jiuhao Chen is based at Ningshan County Hospital, Shaanxi, China.

Jianmin Gao is based in the School of Public Policy and Administration at Xi'an Jiaotong University, Xi'an, China.

Alex Jingwei He is the Associate Head of the Department of Asian and Policy Studies at the Hong Kong Institute of Education. He co-edits the *Journal of Asian Public Policy*. He specializes in health policy and reforms with particular reference to East Asia.

Dan Hu is based at the China Center for Health Development Studies at Peking University, Beijing, China.

Xiaoyun Liu is based in the China Center for Health Development Studies at Peking University, Beijing, China.

Qingyue Meng is a leading expert in health policy and economics. He has widely published in many prestigious journals. He is the Dean of the School of Public Health at Peking University, Beijing, China, and a key health policy advisor to the Chinese government.

Jay Pan is based in the West China School of Public Health at Sichuan University, Chengdu, China.

Yishan Pan is based at Zhenping County Hospital, Shaanxi, China.

Jiwei Qian is a Research Fellow in the East Asian Institute at the National University of Singapore. His research interests include health economics, political economy and development economics.

Kerry Ratigan is an Assistant Professor in the Department of Political Science at Amherst College, Massachusetts, USA.

Yanfang Su is based in the Department of Global Health and Population in the School of Public Health at Harvard University, Cambridge, Massachusetts, USA.

Sen Tian is based in the Research Institute of Economics and Management at Southwestern University of Finance and Economics, Chengdu, China.

Chunxiao Wang is based in the School of Government at Sun Yat-Sen University, Guangzhou, China.

Shaolong Wu is a Researcher in the School of Public Health at Sun Yat-Sen University, Guangzhou, China.

Qiang Yu is based at the Ankang Municipal Development and Reform Commission, Ankang, China.

Guoying Zhang is based in the School of Public Administration at South China Normal University, Guangzhou, China.

Minmin Zhang is based at the China Center for Health Development Studies at Peking University, Beijing, China.

Shichao Zhao is based at the Center for Health Management and Policy at Shandong University, Jinan, China.

Qin Zhou is based in the National School of Development at Peking University, Beijing, China.

Zhiying Zhou is based in the School of Public Health at Xi'an Jiaotong University Health Science Center, Xi'an, China.

Zhongliang Zhou is based in the School of Public Policy and Administration at Xi'an Jiaotong University, Xi'an, China.

INTRODUCTION

An interim interdisciplinary evaluation of China's national health care reform: emerging evidence and new perspectives

Alex Jingwei He[a] and Qingyue Meng[b]

[a]Department of Asian and Policy Studies, The Hong Kong Institute of Education, Hong Kong; [b]China Center for Health Development Studies, Peking University, Beijing, China

Five years have elapsed since the Chinese government unveiled its ambitious health care reform in 2009. A critical juncture in the reform process has been reached and it is time to assess its performance to date in order to inform the next phase of the reform. This article serves as both a review of important studies in the English language literature and the editorial of a special issue titled 'An interim interdisciplinary evaluation of China's national health care reform'. Comprising of six individual research articles, this issue represents a rigorous interim appraisal of the reform from an interdisciplinary perspective. The key message of this issue is threefold. First, social insurance is not the silver bullet for China's health care reform; a revamp is needed to provide better financial protection and to facilitate the move to strategic purchasing. Second, orchestrated reform of the delivery system is needed to address the root causes of rapid cost escalation and vast inefficiency: provider payment reform is the key. Third, in managing the reform process, strategic attention must be given to the dynamic interaction of institutions and incentives. Good governance matters.

1. Introduction

Five years have elapsed since the Chinese government announced its ambitious health care reform programme in 2009. The fact that both the United States and China unfolded their gigantic national health care reforms almost simultaneously is reflective of the daunting health policy challenges that most national governments are grappling with. Skyrocketing costs and continuous demand for quality improvement best describe the thorny problems testing the wisdom of policy-makers. While Obamacare has barely survived the obstruction from Congress and remains controversial, its Chinese counterpart has concluded its first phase at a fairly smooth pace. Having had three trillion RMB invested into it within five years,[1] this landmark reform stands out as one of the biggest health policy interventions in modern history in terms of both scale and scope. Is this reform a success? One can hardly reach a definitive conclusion given the multidimensionality of the reform programme and the much longer time span needed to assess its effects. But what is certain is that the ongoing reform has been transforming a system that affects the health of 1.3 billion people in a dramatic manner. An interim evaluation will be helpful at this critical stage when the Chinese government is searching for solid evidence to improve the current reform agenda.

This special issue presents a rigorous interim evaluation of the reform by a group of scholars from various research fields based in Asia and the United States. As guest editors, the authors of this introductory article purposefully defined the interdisciplinary nature of the issue at the beginning for two reasons. First, while health policy studies are inherently multidisciplinary undertakings, the approach of health economics has traditionally played a dominant role. Recent years have seen an increased recognition of the value of interdisciplinary voices. Contributions from the fields of political science, sociology, public administration and political economy have greatly enriched people's understanding of the intrinsic complexities of health policy (Hsiao 2007, Ho 2010, Duckett 2011, He 2012, Huang 2013, Cheng 2014, Dong *et al.* 2014). In this issue, we seek to create an intellectual platform conducive for the investigation of a huge and complex policy reform from complementary perspectives.

Second, health policy makers looking for practical advice often get caught between theoretically prescribed solutions and peculiar local constraints. The twists and turns of reforms in many countries repeatedly echo what Marc Roberts and his colleagues said:

> Because money flows and incentives are so important in understanding any health system, we make extensive use of economic analysis. But we also believe that incentives alone do not explain everything... .We argue that attention to technical issues alone will never allow a reformer to fully understand and be effective in real situation. (Roberts *et al.* 2002, p. vi)

We thus provide the policy-makers/reformers of China and other transitional economies with a set of analytically rigorous evidence as well as with prescriptions on several integral dimensions of the reform. This special issue aims to facilitate vigorous policy learning and policy transfer through evidence-based results.

This introductory article proceeds as follows. Section 2 briefly reviews the recent history of China's health care reform and outlines its key goals, priorities and strategies. In Section 3, we critically survey the English language literature since 2009, aiming to review the important research findings that have emerged since the commencement of the reform. Section 4 outlines the purposes, central arguments and policy implications of the six individual articles in this issue, highlighting the new perspectives they offer. Section 5 concludes the article.

2. China's health care reform: a brief overview

The Chinese health system's fall from being an internationally revered model to one ranked at the bottom by the World Health Organization was fast and dramatic. The course of its deterioration was not unique but rather followed the general path observed in most transitional economies. Government funding for health first dwindled because of the poorly performing state economy and the crowd-out effect from other areas that were competing for limited fiscal resources (Hsiao 1995). The health care financing system was drastically weakened following structural changes in the economy. Within a rather short period of time, the large majority of residents who had been insured under the command economy became unprotected. Neither the utilization nor the accessibility of care was improved, and for the vulnerable population, financial barriers were elevated (Hu *et al.* 1999, Gao *et al.* 2001). Quality of service and access to care were further undermined because the delivery system built up in the command economy remained largely inefficient. Hospitals and health workers soon found themselves trapped between social obligations and new economic incentives. The typical government delivery model was transformed into a market-oriented system characterized by high out-of-pocket payments and profit-driven providers (Gu 2001, Ma *et al.* 2008).

Such narratives largely reflect what the East European and Asian transitional econo-mies experienced in the last two decades of the twentieth century, but the Chinese story is more complex. First, unable to adequately finance health care, the government allowed hospitals to heavily rely on user charges for financial survival. The share of government subsidies in the total revenue for public hospitals dropped significantly from 50% to 60% to less than 10%. Generating more than 90% of their income from user fees, public hospitals became fully motivated to draw deeper from patients' pockets (Liu and Hsiao 1995, Yip and Hsiao 2008). This perverse incentive was exacerbated by various forms of bonus schemes that tied physicians' incomes with their performance in terms of revenue generation (Likun *et al.* 2000, Liu and Mills 2003). Medical ethics largely evaporated.

Second, the inappropriate incentives were further reinforced by a defective fee sche-dule that set the prices for basic medical services and pharmaceuticals low while leaving expensive procedures, tests and drugs with a higher profit margin. Intended to improve access to basic care, this scheme encouraged providers to switch to profitable items but skimp on basic cost-effective services (Liu *et al.* 2000). The well-known consequence of this system has been the pervasive over-prescription of drugs and high-tech diagnostics tests, leading to massive inefficiencies and a heavy financial burden on patients (Reynolds and McKee 2009, 2011, Currie *et al.* 2011). Hospitals generate half of their revenue from selling drugs. Compounding the over-provision of care is the reliance on fee-for-service as the method for paying providers (Hu *et al.* 2008).

Third, a variety of inappropriate incentives has led to the irrational expansion of tertiary curative services but a neglect of primary and preventive care that underpinned the marvellous health achievements in Mao's era. Dazzling infrastructural development and long queues in big hospitals as well as fierce medical arm races stand in stark contrast to the underfunded and underutilized primary facilities. A referral system and gatekeeping exist in name only. A fragmented and uncoordinated health delivery system has further contributed to cost-ineffective care (Yip and Hsiao 2008, 2014).

The aspects outlined above are merely part of the misaligned incentives embedded in the Chinese health system since the 1980s. The consequences, *kanbing nan* (expensive access to care) and *kanbing gui* (medical impoverishment), have sparked vast public discontent with the health system. Behind this situation is the double-digit escalation of China's health care expenditure, which climbed to 5.36% of the country's GDP in 2012 (see Figure 1).

The landmark health care reform plan announced in early 2009 was the product of five years of deliberation, with extensive participation from academics and stakeholders. Remarkably, a handful of prestigious internal as well as external think tanks – including the World Bank, WHO, Peking University and Fudan University – were invited to provide independent reform proposals. The heated debate between 'the government approach' and 'the market approach' was eventually settled on a mixed version that guarantees a level of basic universal health care while permitting market space to meet additional demands (Ho 2010). Kornreich *et al.* (2012) contend that this participatory consultation process embo-died a major transition of policy-making in China and contributed to better governance by generating popular expectations for inclusion and responsiveness.

At the heart of the reform lies the reassertion of the state's role in health care. The stated overarching goal is to assure that every citizen has equal access to affordable and equitable care by 2020. The reform plan specifically identified five key areas: expanding the coverage of social insurance schemes, establishing a national essential medicines system, advancing public hospital reforms, improving the primary care system and increasing the equality and availability of public health services. An additional 850 billion

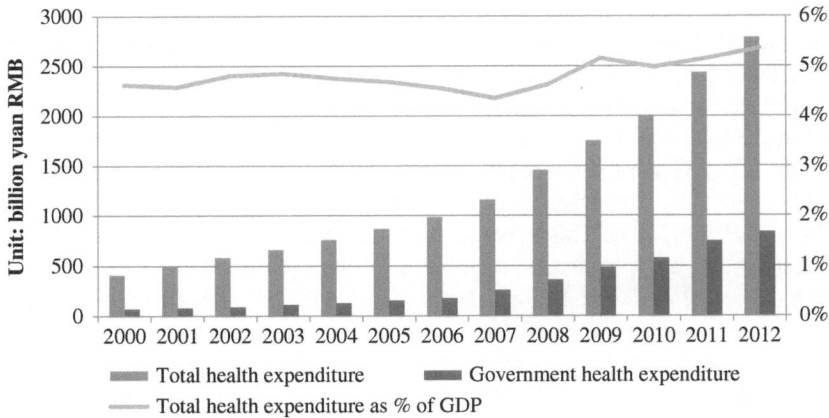

Figure 1.   Government health expenditure, total health expenditure and its share in GDP, 2000–2012.
Source: 2013 China Health Statistical Yearbook, Beijing (online edition), http://www.nhfpc.gov.cn/htmlfiles/zwgkzt/ptjnj/year2013/index2013.html.

RMB (approximately US$125 billion) was to be spent in the first phase of the reform from 2009 to 2011. A high-ranking central steering committee headed by the then vice-premier Li Keqiang was established to coordinate the reform. The entire subnational administrative hierarchy has also been mobilized to develop local adaptations of the national reform formula, and local governments have been encouraged to embark on policy experimentations.

3. Review of recent literature

This section surveys the abundant literature published in recent years examining China's health care reform in order to synthesize the emerging evidence for an interim evaluation. We included both empirical quantitative studies and qualitative analyses published after 2009 in English, but so as not to miss significant insights, we did not exclude important contributions dating back to a couple of years before the reform commenced. We targeted major international journals and other forms of publications in the fields of health economics, health policy, political science, public administration and China studies. Admittedly, the most up-to-date analyses may not be available yet given the longer production cycle of international journals, while those published after 2009 may not necessarily have used data reflecting the situation since the reform. The review is anchored to four strategic aspects of the reform: (1) health insurance and its impacts on utilization and health care costs, (2) the containment of health care expenditure and the reform of how providers are paid, (3) the development of primary health care, and (4) the pilot of public hospital reform.

3.1. Health insurance, utilization and costs

Using the data from the 2003, 2008 and 2011, National Health Service Surveys, Meng *et al.* (2012) found a rapid increase in the coverage of social insurance schemes, namely Urban Employees Basic Medical Insurance (UEBMI), Urban Residents Basic Medical Insurance (URBMI) and the New Cooperative Medical Scheme (NCMS). As of 2011,

95.7% of the population, or about 1.28 billion people, were insured, representing a remarkable progress in contrast to the situation in 2003 when only 10% of the Chinese population was covered by any type of risk pooling programme. This improvement can largely be attributed to the strong political will of the central leadership, substantive government subsidies and the high mobilization capacity of the administrative machinery.

As predicted, the most significant impact observed has been the increased utilization of health services, reflecting eased access to care. In parallel with the marked increase in outpatient visits, hospital admissions more than doubled between 2003 and 2011; the effect was most significant in rural areas (Meng *et al.* 2012). Increased utilization has also been reported in many other findings based on empirical data from various regions; the effect was most remarkable in prenatal services and delivery care (Lei *et al.* 2009, Wagstaff *et al.* 2009, Long *et al.* 2010, Li and Zhang 2013, Wang *et al.* 2014a).

Having brought nearly one billion people back under financial protection, the NCMS has been the most extensively researched aspect of China's health care reform in the past decade. While, in general, the NCMS has been found to be associated with increased service utilization, a noticeable disparity exists across regions and medical sectors. For instance, the study by Yu *et al.* (2010a) in Shandong and Ningxia found that although inpatient service utilization had increased, the effect was significant only for high-income groups, suggesting that middle- and low-income enrollees may not have benefited. Moreover, compared with inpatient services, outpatient service utilization had not seen proportionate increase. Another case study in Gansu Province also found that people with NCMS coverage were less likely to have outpatient visits (Li and Zhang 2013). This disparity could mainly be explained by the fact that the NCMS, as a highly decentralized system, gives local governments vast autonomy in system design. Thus, varying degrees of local government subsidies for premiums, levels of coinsurance and deductibles and even reimbursement procedures may lead to this outcome. Yet it is noteworthy that most of the case studies published thus far were based in less developed regions, while studies analysing the implementation of the NCMS in richer localities are scant.

With the expansion of insurance coverage, the average percentage of inpatient costs reimbursed by insurance schemes rose sharply from 14.4% in 2003 to 46.9% in 2011 (Meng *et al.* 2012). This hoped-for result is also in line with the declining percentage of out-of-pocket expenditure in total health spending (see Figure 2). However, Zhang and Liu (2014) analysed secondary data and demonstrated that the affordability of personal health care has hardly improved since the reform as the share of out-of-pocket payments in disposable personal income has continued to rise. In other words, the reform has not yet made significant progress in its professed goal of providing affordable care. This conclusion is supported by most recent empirical analyses that have demonstrated the very limited effects of social insurance, particularly the NCMS, in reducing people's out-of-pocket burden, predominantly because of ever-increasing health care costs.

Case studies in Linyi, Shandong Province (Sun *et al.* 2009, 2010) and Liaoning Province (Wang *et al.* 2014b) and a comparative analysis of Shandong and Ningxia (Yu *et al.* 2010a) – all revealed that heavy out-of-pocket payments remain a severe financial burden for rural households. Studies using nationally representative survey data also found no evidence of decreased out-of-pocket expenditure, while catastrophic diseases and medical impoverishment remain high risks for poor households (Lei *et al.* 2009, Wagstaff *et al.* 2009, Yip and Hsiao 2009a, Yang *et al.* 2013, Cheng *et al.* 2014).

The reason for this worrisome trend is threefold. First, high deductibles and co-payments, low reimbursement rates and unsupportive claim procedures have created major barriers. These barriers are compounded by the low portability of insurance

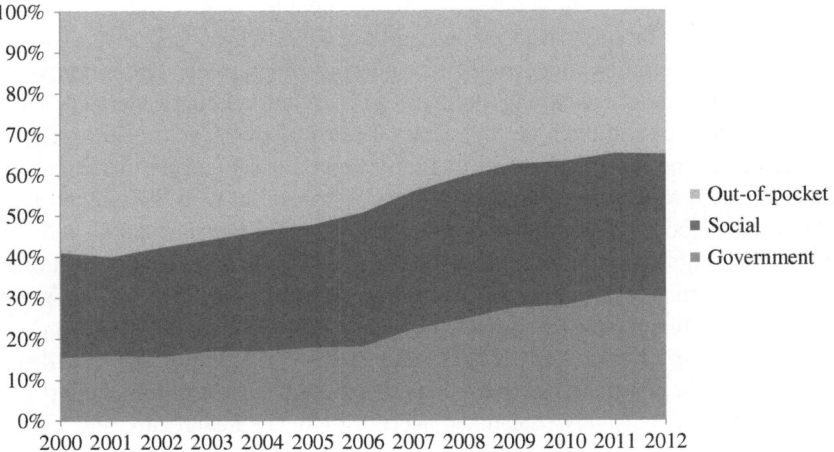

Figure 2. Composition of total health expenditure, 2000–2012.
Source: 2013 China Health Statistical Yearbook, Beijing (online edition), http://www.nhfpc.gov.cn/htmlfiles/zwgkzt/ptjnj/year2013/index2013.html.

benefits, an additional hurdle for the vast floating population (Mou *et al.* 2009, Peng *et al.* 2010). Second, the NCMS in most localities is biased against outpatient services and covers few costs other than those incurred in inpatient care. Yang (2014) noted that despite the financial protection offered by the NCMS, expensive outpatient services constitute the primary reason for sustained medical impoverishment and inequality. The third and the most important reason behind the continued expensive access to care is uncurbed cost inflation.

Insurance-induced demand and the resultant cost explosion are not new. Total costs tend to surge because insurance encourages the insured to seek care when sick. Wagstaff and Lindelow (2008) have already observed that insurance increases the risk of high and catastrophic spending in the UEBMI scheme. When it is compounded with a low benefit level and supplier induced demand, insurance is often found to aggravate the out-of-pocket burden. Wagstaff *et al.* (2009) and Yang and Wu (2014) illustrated that the NCMS has also resulted in people receiving more expensive health care. An empirical study in Guangdong Province used four common diseases as tracers and found that hospitalization costs were systematically higher among insured patients than among uninsured patients as the insured tended to have considerably longer lengths of stay (Pan *et al.* 2009). Other supporting evidence includes the excessively higher incidence of Caesarean sections for the insured, albeit this mode of delivery is prevalent in China (Bogg *et al.* 2010, Long *et al.* 2010, 2012), and inappropriate hospital admissions partly promoted by flawed social insurance designs (Zhang *et al.* 2014b).

3.2. Cost containment and payment reforms

One of the most daunting challenges for the ongoing reform is containing the rapid inflation of health care costs, without which the huge financial resources injected into the reform will hardly help achieve the reform goals but rather will further fuel the massive inefficiencies that are already rather pervasive in the health system (Yip and Hsiao 2008). As the continuous escalation of costs is deeply rooted in a wide range of misaligned incentives embedded in the system, many new initiatives, all aimed at certain aspects of the existing incentive structure, have emerged in local pilots. While the majority of the experiments target the hard economic incentives, particularly those on the supply side, a special type of intervention was adopted in Fujian Province. Here, the local health bureaus tightened the administrative screws and required public hospitals to squeeze excessive profits. By setting ceilings for cost increases, the bureaus sought to slow down the upward spiral of cost escalation. However, as expected, both hospitals and frontline physicians complied ostensibly while engaging in a variety of opportunistic behaviours to defend their economic interests (He and Qian 2013). The case of Fujian suggests that administrative campaigns alone are unable to curb unnecessary care.

There is a wide agreement that fee-for-service, the dominant method of paying providers in China, is cost inflationary and responsible for the galloping medical costs (Hu *et al.* 2008). A number of successful experiments involving a switch from a fee-for-service budget to capitation, case-mix or global budget have been found to be associated with reduced average costs and/or length of stay (Yip and Eggleston 2001, 2004, Zhang 2010, Gao *et al.* 2014). The World Bank (2010a) has provided a comprehensive review of fresh evidence from local reforms published in Chinese. Most experiments have yielded marked effects in cost containment, as predicted by theories. Yet a major weakness of the existing literature is that few studies have thoroughly examined whether payment reforms have compromised quality of care.

Several salient behavioural responses of providers have been found following the switch to alternative payment systems. For instance, Zhang's study in Shanghai, using difference-in-difference strategies, discovered that hospitals engaged in several opportunistic behaviours in reaction to a diagnostic-related groups (DRG) pilot in order to safeguard profits. Specifically, hospitals were found to be reducing the length of stay of patients with the target disease but not reducing outlays. More importantly, hospitals were found to be engaging in cost-shifting tactics in which they raised outlays on uninsured patients to compensate for reduced revenues from insured patients (Zhang 2010).

Another empirical investigation on a capitation reform in Changde, Hunan Province found a marked reduction in inpatient out-of-pocket costs and length of stay but no discernible effect in terms of total inpatient costs and the drug–cost ratio. Further examination revealed cross-sector cost shifting: hospitals responding to the capitation reform by increasing the volume of outpatient care, which was still paid for by the fee-for-service method (Gao *et al.* 2014).

Cost shifting appears to be the chief strategy to which providers resort in reaction to payment reforms. In a case study in Beijing, Jian *et al.* (2009) observed that following a per diem reimbursement reform, while the average length of stay decreased, daily outlays actually increased. They illuminated the puzzle by disentangling the complex incentives within Chinese public hospitals. Although hospital managers are driven by the administrative pressure imposed by government and by economic incentives from the market, they also have to respond to internal appeals from staff. Jian and Guo elucidated that this constitutes a form of internal contract between hospital and staff, with the latter's pursuit mainly resting on safeguarding bonus income. This explanation echoes He and Qian's (2013) analysis in Fujian, which argued that any policy intervention that might affect frontline physicians' tangible economic interests will be resisted by their opportunistic behaviours. Hence, the effects of payment reforms will be undermined unless they proceed in tandem with the realignment of internal incentives.

The concept of pay-for-performance (P4P) has gained prominence in recent years and has been incorporated into a few newly launched payment reforms in China. Wang *et al.*

(2011b) reported an experiment in Guizhou Province that introduced a salary-plus-bonus payment method for village doctors in lieu of fee for service and removed the incentives for over-prescribing medications. The analysis showed that both outpatient costs and drug spending had dropped, but doctors increased non-drug services such as injections and gained more incentives to refer patients to hospital care, which in turn increased total health care costs. A more encouraging result has come from a natural experiment in Ningxia Province, where an intervention targeted at primary care providers combined capitation with pay-for-performance incentives. Both antibiotic prescriptions and total outpatient spending were found to have declined without major adverse effects on other aspects of care (Yip *et al.* 2014). All of the evidence accumulated so far, albeit new and slim, has clearly demonstrated the potential of pay-for-performance strategies.

3.3. Primary health care

A key objective of the current reform is to revive China's once envied primary health system that unfortunately deteriorated during the country's market transition. Until the recent reform, underfunding, low utilization, poor staff qualifications, inefficiency and low patient satisfaction had plagued the system (Bhattacharyya *et al.* 2011). The current primary care reform was designed to improve access, quality and efficiency through a comprehensive set of measures, including a large injection of funds, better training and other supportive policies. Ultimately, the strengthening of primary care is expected to help rebuild a well-structured delivery system (Wang *et al.* 2011a).

There has so far been a paucity of empirical evaluations of primary care reforms. Among the few published studies, results are mixed. Liu *et al.* (2014) investigated the reform in Anhui Province and presented fairly positive results in terms of cost containment, increased government funding, improved personnel structure, reduced drug spending and increased utilization, but the descriptive nature of this study did not allow it to account for confounding factors. Another case study employed more rigorous methods to analyse the pre- and post-reform data on community health centres (CHCs) in Beijing. The analysis found low utilization, suggesting that primary facilities still fail to attract patients despite heavy investment. The majority of patients still regard CHCs as places for drug dispensing and prescription refills (Zhang *et al.* 2011). In another case study in Wuhan, Hubei Province, Zhang *et al.* (2014a) found rather low social recognition of CHCs, with the majority of people still preferring secondary or tertiary facilities when seeking care. Similar findings were also reported in Dalian, Liaoning Province (Dib *et al.* 2010). These findings suggest the limited impact of the reform in altering demand-side incentives. Despite their stated role as the first point of care, the utilization of community health services remains low (Bhattacharyya *et al.* 2011).

The supply-side reform mainly seeks to change the behavioural patterns of primary facilities – with government investment – towards the more efficient and equitable provision of care. Salary reform has been introduced in most localities, with health professionals in grassroots facilities becoming fully salaried staff. The intention of this salary reform is to dissolve profit pressures and enable staff to focus on providing quality public health services and appropriate medical treatments (Yu *et al.* 2011). However, it has generated rather polarized feedback across regions because although it has substantively increased the income level of health workers in poor areas, health workers in many rich areas have actually seen their real income drop. This has not only eroded staff morale but also created a further obstacle in staff recruitment (Zhou *et al.* 2014).

Commonly known as the 'separation of revenue and cost', another widely adopted key initiative strives to remove primary facilities' incentives for providing unnecessary care by delinking income and expenditure, with the shortfall compensated by government subsidies (Li and Yu 2011). As expected, the system has pulled down drug expenditure and the drug–cost ratio in most primary facilities but not necessarily overall costs due to cost shifting (You *et al.* 2011). Moreover, this policy has had a negative impact on the morale of primary health workers due to the reduction of their incomes. The central government is now in the midst of addressing the issues that have surfaced. However, it may take longer to see a rigorous analysis in the English language literature.

In parallel with the primary care reform, the newly established National Essential Medicines System (NEMS) also principally targets primary facilities. The disorder in the Chinese pharmaceutical market is well known. Particularly notorious is the price mark-up policy that allowed a 15–25% profit margin for drugs dispensed in health care facilities (Yu *et al.* 2010b). Coupled with other perverse incentives, this policy greatly motivated the irrational use of prescriptions, especially those involving the abuse of antibiotics. The NEMS aims to increase the availability of cost-effective medicine, ensure the quality of medicine and promote the rational use of medications. This centralized system regulates a wide spectrum of activities, including the selection, production, supply, use, pricing and payment of essential medicines. The system includes a new National Essential Medicines List, with zero price mark-ups, for primary care institutions. The central purpose is to promote the rational use of medicine and remove providers' incentives for over-prescription.

The effects of the NEMS to date, however, have not been completely encouraging. Although the average costs per prescription and total drug costs have declined significantly, as evidenced in case studies (Li *et al.* 2013, Yang *et al.* 2013), the inappropriate use of medications, particularly the over-prescription of antibiotics and injectables, remains prevalent in primary care facilities (Chen *et al.* 2010, Yang *et al.* 2013, Song *et al.* 2014). Other studies have pointed out that the limited range of drugs on the list and the availability of certain drugs have become major concerns for frontline physicians (Chen *et al.* 2010, Tian *et al.* 2012, Zhou *et al.* 2014).

A more comprehensive primary care reform has come from Ningxia Province. Synthesizing both supply-side and demand-side interventions, this reform has sought to improve primary care services by radically altering a wide range of incentives. The NCMS has seen its benefit package reoriented away from inpatient care towards outpatient care, while a tiered reimbursement structure further incentivizes patients to visit primary facilities. The arrangement for paying providers was also changed from fee-for-service to capitation with pay-for-performance incentives. The outcomes thus far are mixed: Although the intended increase in outpatient utilization at village clinics has been achieved through the insurance reform alone, the two interventions in combination have yielded no effect on health care utilization, suggesting that the supply-side intervention has failed to change care-seeking behaviours (Powell-Jackson *et al.* 2014).

The evidence gleaned to date is far from being conclusive, but it is clear that the huge government investment in primary care has not yet been fully translated into increased utilization of affordable quality care and appropriate care-seeking behaviours. The success of primary care reform is ultimately dependent on concerted efforts to deal with certain aspects of the reform such as the training of a large number of competent general practitioners, the provision of supportive insurance reimbursement arrangements, government regulation and accountability (Wang *et al.* 2011a).

3.4. Public hospital reforms

Taking the lion's share in service delivery, public hospitals are the cornerstone of the Chinese health care system. Following the dramatic deterioration of the primary health system during the country's transition to a market economy, the provision of health care in China has become remarkably hospital centred. The absence of proper referral and gate-keeping mechanisms has further weakened coordination within the system, leaving the provision of care fragmented and inefficient (Liu 2004, Yip and Hsiao 2008). All economic incentives point to the competition for and the retention of patients for profit, whereas the considerations of quality of care and cost efficiency have had to take a back seat, leading to long queues and overutilization. As illustrated in the last section, public hospitals in China behave as for-profit entities. Various inappropriate behaviours, including over-prescription and bribe taking, have fuelled social mistrust towards the medical profession and significantly damaged the doctor–patient relationship (He 2014).

Recognizing the challenges in reforming profit-driven hospitals, both Premier Li Keqiang and his predecessor Wen Jiabao stressed that public hospital reform was the 'hard bone' in the comprehensive reform of health care. It has been acknowledged that the highly wasteful delivery system is the perverse engine behind China's skyrocketing health expenditure and that the entire social insurance system would become unsustainable if supply-side reforms fail (Yip and Hsiao 2008). Notwithstanding the central role of public hospital reform, it has been the least understood part of the whole health care reform programme, in part due to its slow progress (Barber *et al.* 2013). Empirical studies on this aspect of health care reform are scant.

The sheer size of China frustrates any one-size-fits-all reform recipe. Nor is it the central government's intention to generalize such ones at the early stage of reform. The government has selected 17 cities to embark on pilots, with considerable autonomy given on programme design. Some pilots are piecemeal reforms, and others with big ambitions have not made the expected progress. A few qualitative interviews with senior government officials have revealed the lack of enthusiasm at local level, primarily due to financial and efficiency concerns (He 2011).

Except for a couple of comprehensive reviews (World Bank 2010b, Barber *et al.* 2013), there are very few studies available on these public hospital pilots in the English language literature. Some major aspects, including payment reforms, separating revenues and costs, and the zero mark-up policy discussed above, all belong to the broad public hospital reform programme. The government has launched other programmes, such as the clinical pathways pilot that seeks to standardize the treatment of common diseases and contain escalating costs. A preliminary assessment, however, suggests the limited effects of these programmes. Profit concerns were found to be still driving the behaviours of both hospitals and physicians, illustrating that the incompatibility of old and new incentives considerably undermines the efficacy of the new reform measures (He and Yang 2015).

The slow progress of the public hospital reform has not allowed us to depict a picture with deeper insights. The embarrassing status quo seems to reflect a tricky policy gridlock where problem A must be solved in order to solve problem B, but problem B requires a solution to problem C, and the solution to problem C depends on finding a solution to problem A (He 2011). The painstaking search for a local reform recipe clearly mirrors both the complexities of the reform itself and the inability of governments to identify an overarching road map. A noteworthy trend lately has been the government's plan to promote the development of private hospitals, in part to nurture competition with their public counterparts and serve the rising needs of the middle- and high-income classes. In a recent article, Yip and Hsiao (2014) warned Chinese policy-makers to be wary about the potential damage that this move could cause. They stressed that privatization at this stage would further erode the delivery system before a primary-care-centred integrated model could be shaped.

4. New perspectives in this special issue

This special issue comprises six individual articles that cover most of the strategic aspects of the reform programme. As stressed above, we aim to comprehensively evaluate the reform by synthesizing the knowledge contributed by multiple research fields, including health economics, political science, public administration and institutional analysis. In this section, we integrate all the individual studies into the broader literature and reform context, highlight their central theses and articulate their theoretical contributions and policy implications.

The first article by Jiwei Qian echoes a growing body of literature that attempts to explain the past failures of China's health care reform from the perspective of governance. Making extensive use of institutional analysis, scholars have attempted to explain the multitude of barriers encountered in health reforms in terms of fundamental governance problems (Ramesh *et al.* 2013). Hsiao (2007), for example, used the agency theory and contended that the dissonance between the pursuits of the principal (top political leaders) and the agent (the health bureaucracy) resulted in difficulties in reform implementation and this had been compounded by the boycott by the *medical axis of power* formed by the health bureaucracy, hospitals and doctors that resists any reforms deemed harmful to their interests. Huang (2013) focused on problems within the central administrative machinery and argued that the buck-passing polity largely explained the poor coordination within the fragmented central bureaucracy that resulted in policy deadlock.

In the first article, Qian examines both horizontal and vertical institutional arrangements within the Chinese bureaucracy, which are found to be unconducive to the appropriate allocation of authority. At the horizontal level, the existing mechanisms of interdepartmental coordination appear less helpful in terms of exchanging support and enforcing bargaining results. The vertical institutional structure built on a performance evaluation system has not yet given local cadres enough incentives to take health reform forward from the back seat. Qian's article further elucidates the respective roles of health administrations, local governments, social insurers and public hospitals in the complex map of institutions. Highlighting the critical importance of relocating authority, this study provides an alternative perspective from which to analyse many ongoing governance reform efforts such as the establishment of an independent regulatory organization to govern public hospitals and the integration of the management of social insurance schemes.

The second article is written by three public administration scholars. Shaolong Wu, Chunxiao Wang and Guoying Zhang respond to a strategic question: has the health care reform improved efficiency? This is a very timely study in view of the rising concerns about the efficiency performance of the enormous financial investment that has been made since the reform commenced. The authors particularly focus on the provinces that played the most significant intermediary role in the execution of the reform. Analysing a panel data set covering the period between 2003 and 2011, this study reports rather grave findings. Despite heavy investment, the additional financial inputs have actually resulted in efficiency losses in both medical care and public health. In addition, regional disparities have widened rather than narrowed.

The results of this study, albeit astonishing, should actually be interpreted with caution. First, the efficiency defined by the authors mainly refers to technical efficiency. Second, this article attributes the decline of technical efficiency primarily to the reduction in the use of advanced technologies and new pharmaceuticals. This is, as a matter of fact, the exact change desired by reformers given the pervasive abuse of high-tech procedures and expensive drugs in the Chinese health system. As stressed by the authors, more efficient allocation of resources should be built on more scientific payment methods.

The third article contributed by three health economists examines the inequality of social health insurance in China, an issue with critical policy implications. Sen Tian, Qin Zhou and Jay Pan made extensive use of economic analysis and found that the current flat premium structure of major social insurance schemes has actually resulted in an unintended situation in which the poor cross-subsidize the rich. Because of low benefits, high co-payments and deductibles, and the varying degree of elasticity, the benefits of health insurance are unevenly distributed across high-income and low-income groups. In spite of having coverage, low-income groups in fact get less benefits. The authors thus propose an unfairness index to measure the inequality of insurance programmes. Income-adjusted premiums are also recommended to mitigate the apparent inequality.

This study renews the discussion on reforming China's social health insurance system. It has long been acknowledged that the fragmented insurance system needs to be integrated in order to equalize entitlements for all citizens and allow a powerful single purchaser to control provider behaviours (Ramesh et al. 2013). Others have made the criticism that the conservative nature of the social insurance bureaucracy has made it preoccupied with the avoidance of financial risks for the insurance funds but less active in taking aggressive measures to alleviate the out-of-pocket burden, as evidenced by the enormous unspent surplus of insurance pools (Hsiao 2007, Yip and Hsiao 2008). Critics also point to the limited managerial capacity of health insurance agencies (Yan et al. 2011). This article sheds new light on the recalibration of the premium rate and its economic consequences for equality. Its recommendations are of high policy relevance.

The fourth article is written by a political scientist. In this study, Kerry Ratigan seeks to answer an interesting research question: Why has China's experimentalist approach, which has been successful in promoting economic growth, not produced good outcomes in health care? Policy experimentation in a highly decentralized system constitutes a salient feature of the governance style of the Chinese party-state. Strengthening policy adaptability by allowing subnational variation has been the key logic driving health policy implementation (Wang 2011). The abundance of empirical evidence received thus far, however, portrays a rather mixed picture, especially in rural areas. While the NCMS has swiftly covered the majority of peasants within a fairly short period of time, high catastrophic payments and inefficient service delivery have largely remained. The author employed both a quantitative survey and qualitative in-depth interviews to investigate rural health reform in three representative provinces. The findings presented largely reinforce those of other quantitative studies, including villagers' dissatisfaction with the NCMS reimbursement rate, the rapid increase in costs and inadequate services.

While, in general, these findings are hardly new, the contribution of this article lies in its efforts in explaining the notable limitations of experimentalism in China's rural health reforms. The author argues that initial conditions explain the observed regional variation, with poorer provinces having developed a style of governance that is not conducive to experimental policy-making. The incentive structure embedded in the administrative system also serves to impede effective rural health reform. This article sheds new light on the role played by governance and public administration in implementing health reforms at the local level.

Written by Xiaoyun Liu and colleagues, the fifth article investigates the progress of primary health care in this round of comprehensive reforms. In global efforts on health system strengthening (HSS), primary health care has been increasingly recognized as vital to ensure equity, accessibility and efficiency and conducive to cost containment (WHO 2008). It is also seen as a key recipe for overhauling China's crumbling health system. The ongoing reform has put tremendous resources into strengthening the primary health system, especially in rural areas.

This article used both primary and secondary data to examine the progress. Albeit descriptive, this study conducted in three representative provinces provides a very timely update on the situation of township health centres and village clinics, the major providers of health services in the countryside. A series of positive outcomes have been found, such as increased government subsidies and revenues, more training opportunities, more appropriate doctor payment mechanisms and increased utilization of services. Several drawbacks also surfaced from the authors' field investigations, including health workers' continued complaints about low income, staff recruitment and retention difficulties and the quality of staff training programmes. These issues warrant close attention from policy-makers.

The last article is contributed by a group of health policy researchers and practitioners. Zhongliang Zhou and colleagues shift audiences' attention from rural primary care to county hospitals, which provide nearly half of the country's inpatient services. It is well known in the health policy research community that Chinese public hospitals receive half of their income from drug sales, a situation rarely seen in other health systems. This has aggravated the escalation of costs, over-prescription and expensive access to care. A flagship programme of the national health care reform is to abolish the 15–25% price mark-up for pharmaceuticals that has been in place for more than two decades. In the implementation of the NEMS, the zero-mark-up rule has already begun to take effect in community-level facilities. As the policy has not yet been scaled up to secondary or tertiary facilities, little is known about its effect on county hospitals. This study fills the gap.

The authors employed a comparison group-treatment group design and difference-in-difference strategy to evaluate the effects in two county hospitals in Shaanxi Province. They found a marked increase in service provision and total hospital income following the intervention. This suggests that hospitals are resorting to increasing both inpatient and outpatient services to make up the shortfalls resulting from the financial losses due to zero mark-up. The authors argue that the increased service volume is an outcome desired by the government because it may suggest improved accessibility. This study provides important evidence for policy-makers regarding the potential effect of the zero-mark-up policy when implemented in secondary providers.

5. Concluding remarks

Needless to say, the reform has produced laudable achievements in the past five years; particularly impressive is the rapid expansion of insurance coverage. Yet, as China is moving into the 'deep water zone' phase of health reform, more fundamental deficiencies of the system must be addressed in an orchestrated fashion. A series of tentative conclusions can be drawn from the received wisdom of the emerging literature as well as from the new evidence presented in this special issue.

First and foremost, social insurance is not the silver bullet for China's health care reform. Financial protection will continue to be limited if the rapid escalation of health care costs remains unharnessed. A major elevation of benefit standards is also needed in order to better shield the insured population against catastrophic medical spending. However, the fragmentation of insurance and limited managerial capacity have not enabled social health insurance to fully unleash its potential. The creation of a capable and prudent third-party purchaser is of strategic importance in the system's march towards strategic purchasing (Xu and Van Deven 2009, Yip and Hsiao 2009b).

Second, despite the evidence of insurance-induced demands, the root causes of China's double-digit cost escalation stem from the inefficient delivery system. Realigning the perverse incentives is a formidable mission in light of the massive tangible as well as intangible interests involved. The sluggishness of public hospital reform provides clear evidence of the difficulties encountered. While a battery of new initiatives, such as the clinical pathways, the separation of revenue and cost, and salary reform, have produced mixed results, payment reform appears the most promising 'control knob', to use the language of Roberts *et al.* (2002), to realign the fundamental economic incentives. There is a growing consensus that reform of the delivery system ultimately hinges on provider payment reforms (Ramesh and Wu 2009, Yip and Hsiao 2009b).

Third, the mixed outcomes of the many new initiatives, such as the NEMS and primary care reform, reveal the path-dependent nature of health systems. Bloom (2011) has insightfully shown that specific policy interventions are much less important than the way the reform process is managed because any health care reform must ultimately tackle the embedded underlying institutional arrangements if it is to succeed. A constellation of fast-moving as well as slow-moving institutions coexist within the broader institutional environment (Meessen and Bloom 2007). Strategic attention must be given to the compatibility and the interaction between these two categories of institutions that are the ultimate source of the poor reform performance observed thus far.

This relates to the final key message of this special issue: governance matters. Reformers need a holistic vision of good governance encompassing the full range of institutions (formal and informal), incentives (economic, administrative and social), and actors (central and local, public and private). Managing the process of a reform of such magnitude as the ongoing one requires rich interdisciplinary wisdom. This special issue seeks to make a contribution.

Disclosure statement

No potential conflict of interest was reported by the authors.

Funding

This study was supported by the Early Career Scheme of Research Grants Council, the Hong Kong SAR Government [Ref. ECS859213]; the Dean's Research Funding Scheme of the Faculty of Liberal Arts and Social Sciences, the Hong Kong Institute of Education [Ref. ECR2].

Note

1. The People's Daily: 'Government spent three trillion in health care reform in five years', April 9 2014, available at http://finance.people.com.cn/GB/n/2014/0409/c1004-24852932.html, accessed on January 4 2015.

References

Barber, S.L., *et al.*, 2013. The hospital of the future in China: China's reform of public hospitals and trends from industrialized countries. *Health Policy and Planning*. doi:10.1093/heapol/czt023.

Bhattacharyya, O., *et al.*, 2011. Evolution of primary care in China 1997–2009. *Health Policy*, 100, 174–180. doi:10.1016/j.healthpol.2010.11.005

Bloom, G., 2011. Building institutions for an effective health system: lessons from China's experience with rural health reform. *Social Science and Medicine*, 72, 1302–1309.

Bogg, L., *et al.*, 2010. Dramatic increase of Cesarean deliveries in the midst of health reforms in rural China. *Social Science and Medicine*, 70, 1544–1549. doi:10.1016/j.socscimed.2010.01.026

Chen, W., *et al.*, 2010. Availability and use of essential medicines in China: manufacturing, supply and prescribing in Shandong and Gansu Provinces. *BMC Health Services Research*, 10, 211. doi:10.1186/1472-6963-10-211

Cheng, L., *et al.*, 2014. The impact of health insurance on health outcomes and spending of the elderly: evidence from China's new cooperative medical scheme. *Health Economics*. doi:10.1002/hec.3053.

Cheng, J.Y., 2014. Institutions, perceptions and social policy-making of Chinese local governments: a case study of medical insurance policy reforms in Dongguan. *Journal of Asian Public Policy*, 7 (1), 58–70. doi:10.1080/17516234.2013.878973

Currie, J., Lin, W., and Zhang, W., 2011. Patient knowledge and antibiotic abuse: evidence from an audit study in China. *Journal of Health Economics*, 30, 933–949. doi:10.1016/j.jhealeco.2011.05.009

Dib, H.H., *et al.*, 2010. Evaluating community health centers in the city of Dalian, China: how satisfied are patients with the medical services provided and their health professionals? *Health and Place*, 16, 477–488. doi:10.1016/j.healthplace.2009.12.005

Dong, L., Christensen, T., and Painter, M., 2014. Health care reform in China: an analysis of development trends and lack of implementation. *International Public Management Journal*, 17 (4), 493–514. doi:10.1080/10967494.2014.958802

Duckett, J., 2011. Challenging the economic reform paradigm: policy and politics in the early 1980s' collapse of the rural co-operative medical system. *The China Quarterly*, 205, 80–95. doi:10.1017/S0305741010001402

Gao, C., Xu, F., and Liu, G., 2014. Payment reform and changes in health care in China. *Social Science and Medicine*, 111, 10–16. doi:10.1016/j.socscimed.2014.03.035

Gao, J., *et al.*, 2001. Changing access to health services in urban China: implications for equity. *Health Policy and Planning*, 16 (3), 302–312. doi:10.1093/heapol/16.3.302

Gu, E., 2001. Market transition and the transformation of the health care system in urban China. *Policy Studies*, 22 (3–4), 197–215. doi:10.1080/01442870120112692

He, J., 2011. China's ongoing public hospital reform: initiatives, constraints and prospect. *Journal of Asian Public Policy*, 4 (3), 342–349. doi:10.1080/17516234.2011.630228

He, J., 2012. Is the Chinese health bureaucracy incapable of leading healthcare reforms? The case of Fujian Province. *China: An International Journal*, 10 (1), 93–112.

He, J., 2014. The doctor-patient relationship, defensive medicine and overprescription in Chinese public hospitals: evidence from a cross-sectional survey in Shenzhen City. *Social Science and Medicine*, 123, 64–71. doi:10.1016/j.socscimed.2014.10.055

He, J. and Qian, J., 2013. Hospitals' responses to administrative cost-containment policy in urban China: the case of Fujian Province. *The China Quarterly*, 216, 946–969. doi:10.1017/S0305741013001112

He, J. and Yang, W., 2015. Clinical pathways in China: an evaluation. *International Journal of Health Care Quality Assurance*, 28 (3).

Ho, C.S., 2010. Health reform and de facto federalism in China. *China: An International Journal*, 8 (1), 33–62.

Hsiao, W., 1995. The Chinese health care system: lessons for other nations. *Social Science and Medicine*, 41 (8), 1047–1055. doi:10.1016/0277-9536(94)00421-O

Hsiao, W., 2007. The political economy of Chinese health reform. *Health Economics, Policy and Law*, 2, 241–249. doi:10.1017/S1744133107004197

Hu, S., *et al.*, 2008. Reform of how health care is paid for in China: challenges and opportunities. *The Lancet*, 372, 1846–1853. doi:10.1016/S0140-6736(08)61368-9

Hu, T., *et al.*, 1999. The effects of economic reform on health insurance and the financial burden for urban workers in China. *Health Economics*, 8 (4), 309–321. doi:10.1002/(SICI)1099-1050 (199906)8:4<309::AID-HEC440>3.0.CO;2-N

Huang, Y., 2013. *Governing health in contemporary China*. Abingdon: Routledge.

Jian, W., *et al.*, 2009. Does per-diem reimbursement necessarily increase length of stay? The case of a public psychiatric hospital. *Health Economics*, 18, S97–S106. doi:10.1002/hec.1522

Kornreich, Y., Vertinsky, I., and Potter, P.B., 2012. Consultation and deliberation in China: the making of China's health-care reform. *The China Journal*, 68, 176–203. doi:10.1086/666583

Lei, X., *et al.*, 2009. The new cooperative medical scheme in rural China: does more coverage mean more service and better health? *Health Economics*, 18, S25–S46. doi:10.1002/hec.1501

Li, H. and Yu, W., 2011. Enhancing community system in China's recent health reform: an effort to improve equity in essential health care. *Health Policy*, 99, 167–173. doi:10.1016/j.healthpol.2010.08.006

Li, X. and Zhang, W., 2013. The impacts of health insurance on health care utilization among the older people in China. *Social Science and Medicine*, 85, 59–65. doi:10.1016/j.socscimed.2013.02.037

Li, Y., *et al.*, 2013. Evaluation, in three Provinces, of the introduction and impact of China's national essential medicines scheme. *Bulletin of the World Health Organization*, 91, 184–194. doi:10.2471/BLT.11.097998

Likun, P., Legge, D., and Stanton, P., 2000. Policy contradictions limiting hospital performance in China. *Policy Studies*, 21 (2), 99–113. doi:10.1080/713691363

Liu, Q., *et al.*, 2014. Evaluation of the effects of comprehensive reform on primary healthcare institutions in Anhui Province. *BMC Health Services Research*, 14, 268. doi:10.1186/1472-6963-14-268

Liu, X. and Hsiao, W., 1995. The cost escalation of social health insurance plans in China: its implication for public policy. *Social Science and Medicine*, 41 (8), 1095–1101. doi:10.1016/0277-9536(94)00423-Q

Liu, X., Liu, Y., and Chen, N., 2000. The Chinese experience of hospital price regulation. *Health Policy and Planning*, 15 (2), 157–163. doi:10.1093/heapol/15.2.157

Liu, X. and Mills, A., 2003. The influence of bonus payments to doctors on hospital revenue: results of a quasi-experimental study. *Applied Health Economics and Health Policy*, 2 (2), 91–98.

Liu, Y., 2004. China's public health-care system: facing the challenges. *Bulletin of the World Health Organization*, 82 (7), 532–538.

Long, Q., *et al.*, 2010. Utilisation of maternal health care in western rural China under a new rural health insurance system (new cooperative medical system). *Tropical Medicine and International Health*, 15 (10), 1210–1217. doi:10.1111/j.1365-3156.2010.02602.x

Long, Q., *et al.*, 2012. High caesarean section rate in rural China: is it related to health insurance (new cooperative medical scheme)? *Social Science and Medicine*, 75, 733–737. doi:10.1016/j.socscimed.2012.03.054

Ma, J., Lu, M., and Quan, H., 2008. From a national, centrally planned health system to a system based on the market: lessons from China. *Health Affairs*, 27 (4), 937–948. doi:10.1377/hlthaff.27.4.937

Meessen, B. and Bloom, G., 2007. Economic transition, institutional changes and the health system: some lessons from rural China. *Journal of Economic Policy Reform*, 10 (3), 209–231. doi:10.1080/17487870701446033

Meng, Q., *et al.*, 2012. Trends in access to health services and financial protection in China between 2003 and 2011: a cross-sectional study. *The Lancet*, 379, 805–814. doi:10.1016/S0140-6736(12)60278-5

Mou, J., *et al.*, 2009. Health care utilisation amongst Shenzhen migrant workers: does being insured make a difference? *BMC Health Services Research*, 9, 214. doi:10.1186/1472-6963-9-214

Pan, X., *et al.*, 2009. Absence of appropriate hospitalization cost control for patients with medical insurance: a comparative analysis study. *Health Economics*, 18, 1146–1162. doi:10.1002/hec.1421

Peng, Y., *et al.*, 2010. Factors associated with health-seeking behavior among migrant workers in Beijing, China. *BMC Health Services Research*, 10, 69. doi:10.1186/1472-6963-10-69

Powell-Jackson, T., Yip, W.C., and Han, W., 2014. Realigning demand and supply side incentives to improve primary health care seeking in rural China. *Health Economics*. doi:10.1002/hec.3060.

Ramesh, M. and Wu, X., 2009. Health policy reform in China: lessons from Asia. *Social Science and Medicine*, 68, 2256–2262. doi:10.1016/j.socscimed.2009.03.038

Ramesh, M., Wu, X., and He, J., 2013. Health governance and healthcare reforms in China. *Health Policy and Planning*. doi:10.1093/heapol/czs109.

Reynolds, L. and McKee, M., 2009. Factors influencing antibiotic prescribing in China: an exploratory analysis. *Health Policy*, 90, 32–36. doi:10.1016/j.healthpol.2008.09.002

Reynolds, L. and McKee, M., 2011. Serve the people or close the sale? Profit-driven overuse of injections and infusions in China's market-based healthcare system. *The International Journal of Health Planning and Management*, 26, 449–470. doi:10.1002/hpm.1112

Roberts, M.J., *et al.*, 2002. *Getting health reform right*. Oxford University Press.

Song, Y., *et al.*, 2014. The impact of China's national essential medicine system on improving rational drug use in primary health care facilities: an empirical study in four Provinces. *An Empirical Study in Four Provinces, BMC Health Services Research*, 14, 507. doi:10.1186/s12913-014-0507-3

Sun, X., *et al.*, 2009. Catastrophic medical payment and financial protection in rural China: evidence from the new cooperative medical scheme in Shandong Province. *Health Economics*, 18, 103–119. doi:10.1002/hec.1346

Sun, X., *et al.*, 2010. Health payment-induced poverty under China's new cooperative medical scheme in rural Shandong. *Health Policy and Planning*, 25, 419–426. doi:10.1093/heapol/czq010.

Tian, X., Song, Y., and Zhang, X., 2012. National essential medicines list and policy practice: a case study of China's health care reform. *BMC Health Services Research*, 12, 401. doi:10.1186/1472-6963-12-401

Wagstaff, A. and Lindelow, M., 2008. Can insurance increase financial risk? The curious case of health insurance in China. *Journal of Health Economics*, 27 (4), 990–1005. doi:10.1016/j.jhealeco.2008.02.002

Wagstaff, A., *et al.*, 2009. Extending health insurance to the rural population: an impact evaluation of China's new cooperative medical scheme. *Journal of Health Economics*, 28, 1–19. doi:10.1016/j.jhealeco.2008.10.007

Wang, H., Gusmano, M.K., and Cao, Q., 2011a. An evaluation of the policy on community health organizations in China: will the priority of new healthcare reform in China be a success? *Health Policy*, 99, 37–43. doi:10.1016/j.healthpol.2010.07.003

Wang, H., *et al.*, 2011b. An experiment in payment reform for doctors in rural China reduced some unnecessary care but did not lower total costs. *Health Affairs*, 30 (12), 2427–2436. doi:10.1377/hlthaff.2009.0022

Wang, S., 2011. Learning through practice and experimentation: the financing of rural health care. In: S. Heilmann and E.J. Perry, eds. *Mao's invisible hand: the political foundations of adaptive governance in China*. Cambridge, MA: Harvard University Press, 102–137.

Wang, S., *et al.*, 2014a. Comparison of Chinese inpatients with different types of medical insurance before and after the 2009 healthcare reform. *BMC Health Services Research*, 14, 443. doi:10.1186/1472-6963-14-443

Wang, X., *et al.*, 2014b. The effects of China's new cooperative medical scheme on accessibility and affordability of healthcare services: an empirical research in Liaoning Province. *BMC Health Services Research*, 14, 388. doi:10.1186/1472-6963-14-388

WHO, 2008. *World health organization report 2008: primary health care (Now more than ever)*. Geneva: The World Health Organization.

World Bank, 2010a. *Health provider payment reforms in China: what international experience tells us?* Washington, DC: The World Bank.

World Bank, 2010b. *Fixing the public hospital system in China*. Washington, DC: The World Bank.

Xu, W. and Van Deven, W., 2009. Purchasing health care in China: competing or non-competing third-party purchasers? *Health Policy*, 92, 305–312. doi:10.1016/j.healthpol.2009.05.009

Yan, F., *et al.*, 2011. Management capacity and health insurance: the case of the new cooperative medical scheme in six counties in rural China. *The International Journal of Health Planning and Management*, 26, 357–378. doi:10.1002/hpm.1028

Yang, L., *et al.*, 2013. The impact of the national essential medicines policy on prescribing behaviours in primary care facilities in Hubei Province of China. *Health Policy and Planning*, 28, 750–760. doi:10.1093/heapol/czs116

Yang, W., 2014. Catastrophic outpatient health payments and health payment-induced poverty under China's new rural cooperative medical scheme. *Applied Economic Perspectives and Policy*. doi:10.1093/aepp/ppu017

Yang, W. and Wu, X., 2014. Paying for outpatient care in rural China: cost escalation under China's new cooperative medical scheme. *Health Policy and Planning*. doi:10.1093/heapol/czt111.

Yip, W. and Eggleston, K., 2001. Provider payment reform in China: the case of hospital reimbursement in Hainan Province. *Health Economics*, 10 (4), 325–339. doi:10.1002/hec.602

Yip, W. and Eggleston, K., 2004. Addressing government and market failures with payment incentives: hospital reimbursement reform in Hainan, China. *Social Science and Medicine*, 58, 267–277. doi:10.1016/S0277-9536(03)00010-8

Yip, W. and Hsiao, W., 2008. The Chinese health system at a crossroads. *Health Affairs*, 27 (2), 460–468. doi:10.1377/hlthaff.27.2.460

Yip, W. and Hsiao, W., 2009a. Non-evidence-based policy: how effective is China's new cooperative medical scheme in reducing medical impoverishment? *Social Science and Medicine*, 68, 201–209. doi:10.1016/j.socscimed.2008.09.066

Yip, W. and Hsiao, W., 2009b. China's health care reform: a tentative assessment. *China Economic Review*, 20, 613–619. doi:10.1016/j.chieco.2009.08.003

Yip, W. and Hsiao, W., 2014. Harnessing the privatisation of China's fragmented health-care delivery. *The Lancet*, 384, 805–818. doi:10.1016/S0140-6736(14)61120-X

Yip, W., *et al.*, 2014. Capitation combined with pay-for-performance improves antibiotic prescribing practices in rural China. *Health Affairs*, 33 (3), 502–510. doi:10.1377/hlthaff.2013.0702

You, C., *et al.*, 2011. A new financial budgetary system for community health services institutions in China. *The International Journal of Health Planning and Management*, 26, 436–448. doi:10.1002/hpm.1113

Yu, B., *et al.*, 2010a. How does the new cooperative medical scheme influence health service utilization? A study in two Provinces in rural China. *BMC Health Services Research*, 10, 116. doi:10.1186/1472-6963-10-116

Yu, X., *et al.*, 2010b. Pharmaceutical supply chain in China: current issues and implications for health system reform. *Health Policy*, 97, 8–15. doi:10.1016/j.healthpol.2010.02.010

Yu, Y., *et al.*, 2011. What should the government do regarding health policy-making to develop community health care in Shanghai? *The International Journal of Health Planning and Management*, 26, 379–435. doi:10.1002/hpm.1117

Zhang, J., 2010. The impact of a diagnosis-related group-based prospective payment experiment: the experience of Shanghai. *Applied Economics Letters*, 17, 1797–1803. doi:10.1080/13504850903317347

Zhang, L. and Liu, N., 2014. Health reform and out-of-pocket payments: lessons from China. *Health Policy and Planning*, 29, 217–226. doi:10.1093/heapol/czt006

Zhang, P., *et al.*, 2014a. Societal determination of usefulness and utilization wishes of community health services: a population-based survey in Wuhan city, China. *Health Policy and Planning*. doi:10.1093/heapol/czu128

Zhang, X., *et al.*, 2011. Tracking the effectiveness of health care reform in China: A case study of community health centers in a district of Beijing. *Health Policy*, 100, 181–188. doi:10.1016/j.healthpol.2010.10.003

Zhang, Y., *et al.*, 2014b. Current level and determinants of inappropriate admissions to township hospitals under the new rural cooperative medical system in China: a cross-sectional study. *BMC Health Services Research*, 14, 649. doi:10.1186/s12913-014-0649-3

Zhou, X.D., Li, L., and Hesketh, T., 2014. Health system reform in rural China: voices of health workers and service users. *Social Science and Medicine*, 17, 134–141.

Reallocating authority in the Chinese health system: an institutional perspective

Jiwei Qian

East Asian Institute, National University of Singapore, Singapore

Affordability of health care is still a serious concern in China after the health reform in 2009. According to the literature of the economics of organization, allocation of authority in hospitals and social insurance is extremely important for improving affordability. The information structure and the degree of conflicts in tasks within an organization determine the optimal allocation of authority. However, the progress of the governance reform to reallocate the authority is relatively slow during the reform period. This article argues that the slow progress is associated with ineffective coordination among government departments in China. Two institutional reasons are illustrated in this article. First, there is no institutional arrangement to facilitate the horizontal coordination among ministries and bureaus. Second, the performance evaluation system for officials, which mainly addresses the vertical coordination between upper and lower level governments, has unintended consequences for horizontal coordination among local government departments. Future reforms should take into account these institutional aspects.

Introduction

China's most recent set of health reforms have entered their sixth year of implementation in 2014. Between 2009 and 2013, the government expenditure on health reached RMB 3 trillion. More importantly, by the end of 2013, over 95% of Chinese citizens were covered by at least one social health insurance programme. Government health expenditure as a share of total health expenditure increased from 15.5% in 2000 to 30.1% in 2013.[1]

Although the universal coverage of social health insurance has been realized, affordability is still a concern. There has been double-digit annual growth in health expenditure in China for the past 10 years. Total health expenditure has reached RMB 3.16 trillion, which accounts for about 5.6% of gross domestic product (GDP) in 2013,[2] compared to about 4% in 1997 (Figure 1). It is estimated the share of health expenditure in GDP will reach 8.4% by 2030 (Ma *et al.* 2012).

Out-of-pocket payment as a percentage of total health expenditure in 2013 was about 34%. More specifically, health care expenditure for a rural and urban resident reached RMB 513 and 1063 in 2012, respectively, compared to RMB 246 and 786 in 2008.

In the literature of the economics of organization, the affordability issue can be addressed by reforming the governance structure by reallocating authority, including delegating, centralizing and restructuring authority in an organization (Bolton and Dewatripont 2012, Gibbons *et al.* 2012). In principle, the information structure and the

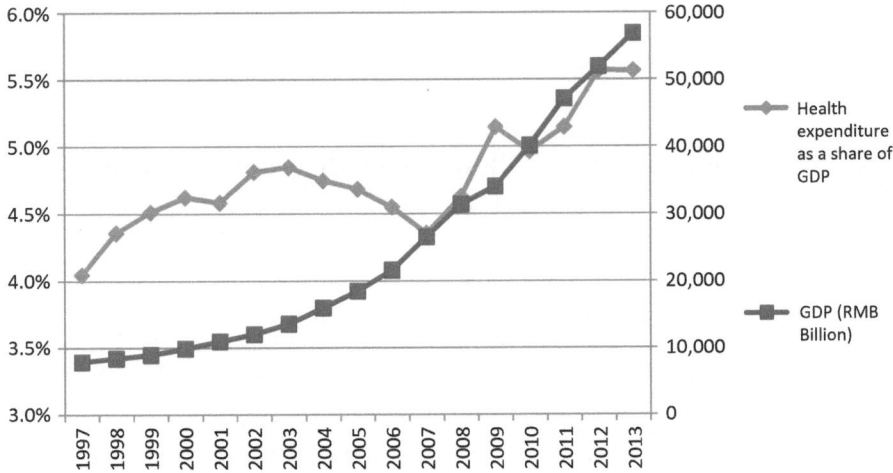

Figure 1. Health expenditure and GDP in China.
Source: China health statistical yearbook, various years & Statistical Communiqué on Health Care and Family Planning Development in China, 2013.

degree of conflicts in tasks within an organization determine the optimal allocation of authority. As long as the incentives conflict between the principal and agents is not too substantial, agents with better access to information shall be granted authority. In this case, authority allocation is an instrument to take advantage of local knowledge/information. In addition, when there are multiple tasks to be fulfilled, authority of dealing with interest-conflicting tasks should be allocated to different agencies. This is to avoid adverse impact of conflict of interests and also to improve accountability because it is easier to measure agencies' performance with focused missions.

For the Chinese health reform, to improve affordability via reallocating authority for health insurance and hospital governance is pivotal since both social insurer and doctors are critical for health care decisions. According to the theory of economics of organization, there are two directions for reallocation authority in the health system. First, information structure matters for an efficient authority allocation. For instance, if a private insurer has better professional expertise of managing risks (i.e. better information), the task to manage social insurance fund may thus be reallocated from social health insurance to a private insurer. Second, authority for of interest-conflicting tasks should be delegated to different agencies. For example, the authority of managing social insurance should be assigned separately to the authority of health service provision, given that these two tasks, the provision and the purchase of health services, are of conflicting interests. It may be more desirable to let local social security bureau, rather than local health bureau, to manage rural social health insurances.

Although there have been some initiatives to reform the health care governance structure since 2009, inefficient allocation of authority is persistent in public hospitals and social insurances. The research question raised by this article is that for what reason, the progress of governance reform to reallocate authority in both public hospitals and social health insurance has been slow since 2009.

The persistence of inefficient authority allocation in the health system is related to an analytical framework in Chinese politics: 'Fragmented Authoritarianism', which claims that the decision-making bodies are fragmented and disjointed among different ministries as well as among different levels of governments (Lieberthal and Oksenberg 1988). This article argues that there are two reasons for the slow progress of governance reform in this fragmented structure. First, while coordination among government departments is necessary for reallocating authority, there is lack of institutions for political actors to exchange support and enforce bargaining results. Second, performance evaluation system for government officials, which is an institutional response to the vertically fragmented structure of policy implementation, has unintended consequences for horizontal coordination among government departments. Officials in local bureaus tend to allocate their efforts on those tasks, which are more rewarding such as promoting economic growth, and they are more likely to be accountable for the local party secretary rather than their ministries.

Policy implication then is to look for a second best solution for reallocation of authority in public hospitals and social insurance, given these constraints of the fragmented structure of policy making and implementation.

This article belongs to a growing literature about political economy of Chinese health reform (Hsiao 2007, Kornreich *et al.* 2012, Huang 2013, Gilli *et al.* 2014). This article differentiates from existing literature in two ways. First, this study interprets the health reform in China through the lens of reallocation of authority defined by the theory of economics of organization. Second, this article highlights that there are institutional reasons associated with the framework of 'Fragmented Authoritarianism', which results in a suboptimal allocation of authority in public hospitals and social health insurances. This article does not simply apply the framework 'Fragmented Authoritarianism' in the context of health reform. Rather, comparing with the committee system in the US congress, this study considers what institutional arrangements are necessary to achieve the coordination among political actors and compliance of bureaucracy. This article shows that when these institutions are absent, the inefficient allocation of authority is persistent in the Chinese health system.

The rest of the article is arranged as follows. The next section reviews status of the recent round of health reform. Then, why reallocation of authority matters and what kind of institutional arrangements can improve efficiency are discussed. Following a discussion on some initiatives in governance reform in the health sector, the difficulty to reallocate authority is shown as a result of institutional constraints in China. Finally, the policy implications and conclusion are drawn.

Progresses and concerns in health reform

Government indeed has taken the lead role in health reform in China. Between 2009 and 2013, one of the most outstanding achievements made by the health reform was the dramatic increase in government health expenditure. According to an official report in April 2013, accumulative government expenditure on health reached RMB 3 trillion during the five-year-period from 2009 to 2013.[3] The share of government expenditure in total health expenditure reached 30.1% in 2013 compared to 15.5% in 2000.

By the end of 2013, over 95% of the 1.36 billion Chinese citizens were covered by at least one social health insurance programme (i.e. Figure 2). In 2014, the government paid subsidies in the amount of RMB 320 for each enrolee under the rural New Cooperative Medical Scheme (NCMS) and Urban Resident health Insurance (URI).[4] Patients' out-of-pocket health expenditure decreased from about 60% of the total expenditure in 2000 to 33.9% in 2013 (see Figure 3).

However, the affordability is still a serious concern after the five-year reform.

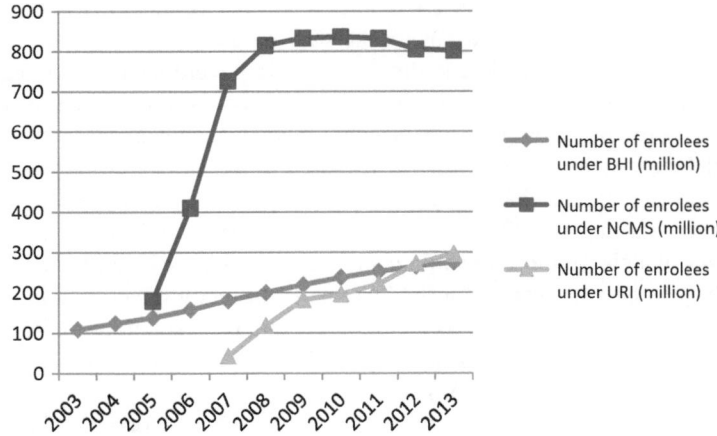

Figure 2. The number of enrolees covered by social insurances.

Source: China health statistical yearbook, various years & Statement of social insurance in China, 2013.

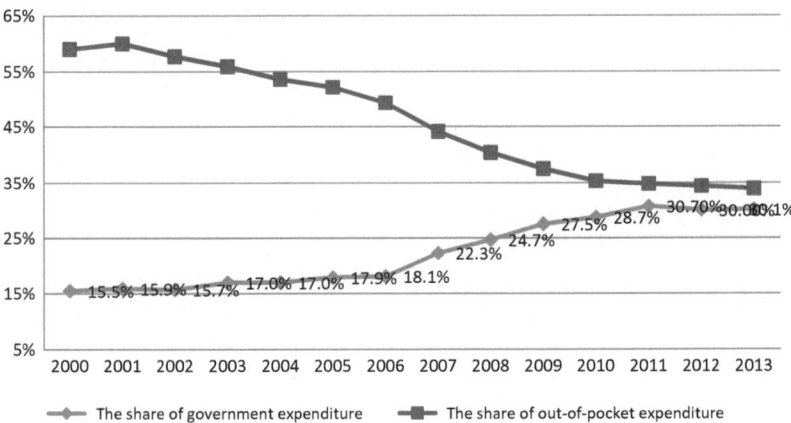

Figure 3. The share of government expenditure/out-of-pocket expenditure in total health expenditure.

Source: China health statistical yearbook, various years & Statistical Communiqué on Health Care and Family Planning Development in China, 2013.

Between 2008 and 2013, out-of-pocket expenditure increased by 12.8% annually in average (Figure 4). Regarding social health insurance, financial coverage is yet insufficient. For example, the upper limit of social health insurance for reimbursement is still low (i.e. about 4–6 times of local average annual income).

Health care providers' profit-seeking behaviour is believed to be the key reason for high health expenditure in China. In particular, public hospitals have the incentive to over-prescribe drugs since public hospitals are entitled to charge a price markup of up to 15% for drug prescription. There is little evidence showing that the incentive structure for public hospital physicians has changed much as yet, and the problems of inappropriate prescription still persist in many places. For instance, a recent study shows that over 60%

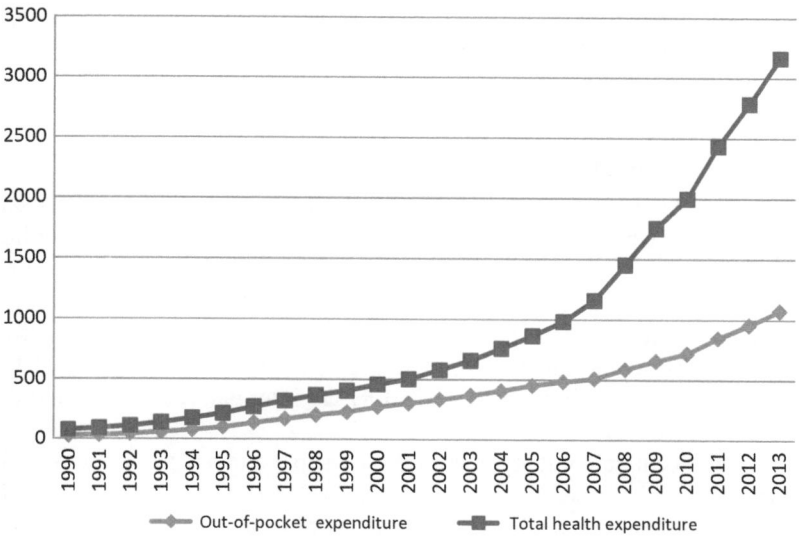

Figure 4. Growth of out-of-pocket expenditure in China.
Source: China health statistical yearbook, various years.

of patients in the sample are prescribed antibiotics that are not compatible with their symptoms. Even for informed patients who understand that antibiotics are not appropriately prescribed in their cases, 39% of these patients have still been prescribed antibiotics (Currie *et al.* 2011). Currie *et al.* (2014) also identify that the over prescription of antibiotics is largely a result of financial incentives of doctors. Figure 5 shows that the share of drug revenue in general hospitals remained at 40% between 2004 and 2012.

The incentives as well as the capacity of social insurers are substantially relevant to address providers' profit-seeking behaviour. Although some localities have started pilot reforms of payment methods (Cheng 2013), the social insurers are short of capacity/ professional training to improve affordability via purchasing health services from providers (Ramesh *et al.* 2014).

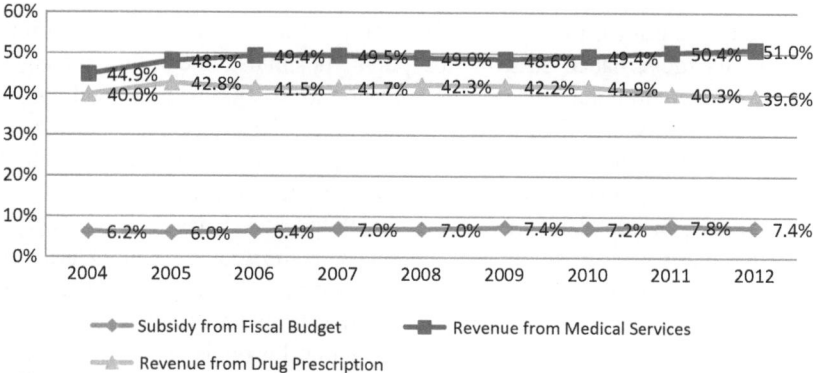

Figure 5. Average share of different sources of revenue in public general hospitals.
Source: China health statistical yearbook, various years.

Also, many local social insurers' objective is merely to balance the budget and not to explore potential payment method reforms to control health service costs.[5]

What is authority and how to allocate authority?

In this section, the implication of authority allocation in public hospitals and social insurance for affordability of health care are going to be discussed. According to the literature of economics of organization, 'authority' is defined with a bundle of decision rights. These decision rights include the power to initiate projects, ratify and approve actions, monitor subordinate's performance as well as exact obedience (Bolton and Dewatripont 2012). As indicated in the literature, to improve efficiency, two determinants of choosing a certain way of allocating authority are information structure and the degree of conflicts in tasks.

First, if the incentive conflict between the principal and agents is not too substantial, the authority should be (re)allocated to the agent who has more information (Laffont and Martimort 2009, Gibbons *et al.* 2012). Some tasks are with more uncertainty and some are more difficult to be measured. In this case, the agent with more/better information is more likely to make efficient decisions. For example, according to recent empirical studies on management performance, managers with MBA training may have more information on what are the best practices to run a firm and may make more efficient decisions (Bloom *et al.* 2014) than those who have no such trainings.

Second, an individual agent may need to fulfil multitasks and the objectives of these tasks may be in conflict with one another. It is likely for an agent to spend more effort on those rewarding tasks and less effort for other tasks. To fulfil all tasks more efficiently, the authority for tasks in conflict may need to be assigned to different agents. For example, many researches interpret the role of the local government in economic development as a firm in the market (Oi 1992). Local economic development is a critical task for local officials in China. However, local officials are also assigned with some other tasks which may be adverse to local economic development. For example, in Wu *et al.* (2013), local officials are not willing to spend on environment infrastructure for pollution control because it is not directly helpful in local GDP growth. It is debated in China now that local environment protection agency should be independent from local government.[6]

Governance reform in the health sector, including various initiatives to reallocate authority such as delegating, centralizing, restructuring authority in public hospitals and social insurance, is critical to improve affordability of health care. These reforms include reorganizing the governance structure of public hospitals, integrating management of social insurance, contracting out insurance service to private insurers, and so on. Given that affordability is associated with behaviour and incentives of public hospitals and social insurers, with various governance reforms to reallocate authority, the affordability issue can be addressed by changing the behaviour of providers and insurers.

For example, for social insurances, an integrated social health insurance plan may have a better bargaining position with hospitals, compared to fragmentarily managed plans. For public hospitals, an independent government agency who regulates public hospitals can address the issue of doctors' incentive to overprescribe drugs.

While the objective of social insurers and public hospitals (i.e. improving financial coverage and delivering more services with quality) may be different from the objective of a firm in the market, the principles for allocating authority in a firm can be applied to the governance of hospitals and social health insurance for two reasons.

First, similar to a firm in the market, hospitals and insurers have multiple tasks, which may be in conflict to one another, and hospitals and insurers also have asymmetric information structure. For example, hospitals need to make sure that their patients are treated properly, while hospitals also need to generate enough financial revenue to sustain daily operations. For social health insurers, one task is to increase coverage and improve affordability, while the other task is to keep budget balanced. The task of local health bureau is associated with service delivery, while the task of social insurers is to provide financial coverage for these services. More and better services delivered imply more expenditure from social insurers. These tasks are in conflict with one another. In addition, for a given task, some agents are informed and some are less well informed. For example, compared to social security bureau, which have more experiences in managing social insurance, local health bureau, who manages rural health insurance, may be less familiar with risk management.

Second, hospitals and insurers, similar to a firm in the market, have incentives to improve efficiency. For example, hospitals are keen to minimize the operation costs to treat more patients, given the quality of health services. Insurers want to keep the health expenditure minimum for a given treatment process.

For the above two reasons, the allocation of authority is relevant to improve affordability in the health sector. The governance reform in public hospitals can address the concerns of conflicting tasks and asymmetric information by reallocating authority. For a long time, local health bureaus regulate and manage the operation of public hospitals (Qian and Blomqvist 2014). However, regulating the health service quality and its price is a task in conflict with the task to manage and operate a hospital. In this case, it is more efficient to allocate the authority of regulating and managing to different agents ('guanban fenkai').

Regarding the reform on social health insurance, information structure is important to determine the allocation of authority. Currently, fragmentarily managed social insurers are short of capacity of managing financial risks. It is better to reallocate authority to private insurers with the authority of managing social insurance since they have better information structure. Similarly, an integrated local social health insurer for rural and urban residents and employees can take advantage of better information since the integrated insurer can access to more sufficient information about demand and utilization of local health services.

Slow progress of governance reforms in social insurances and public hospitals

A number of pilot projects on how to reform governance structure of public hospitals and the social health insurances have been initiated since 2009. The governance reform in public hospitals has taken place in various forms. One way is to reform governance structure within the public hospitals. Public hospitals in Shanghai, Ma'an shan, Kunming and Xiamen have been corporatized by establishing independent board of directors and supervisory board.[7]

Another direction of governance reform is to reorganize the structure of health care service provision. For example, some cities such as Beijing have established a new government agency ('Yi Guan Ju') to regulate public hospitals, and public hospitals in these cities are corporatized.[8] In Shanghai, an independent agency to manage public hospitals (i.e. Shen-Kang Hospital Development Center) is allocated with the authority of operating hospitals, and local health bureau has been allocated the authority of regulating. As a conglomerate with 24 hospitals, this new agency may have better information about demand from patients and can make better investment decisions on infrastructure building and resource planning.[9]

For social insurances, one reform direction is to integrate social health insurance plans. By 2014, there are seven provinces integrating the NCMS and URI.[10] In these provinces, integrated social health insurances are managed by a single government agency. Usually, it is the local social security bureau that manages this integrated social health insurance. The administration cost is saved when these insurance programmes share the same health information system, and redundant investments on the information infrastructure are avoided.[11] In addition, under the integrated plan, insurers are likely to have better information for health care service utilization, and it is more effective for social insurers to purchase health care service.

Another direction of governance reform for social health insurances is to engage with private insurers for improving affordability of health care. In August 2012, a government guideline about the 'Catastrophic medical insurance programme' ('Dabing Yibao') was released.[12] The catastrophic medical insurance programme is a supplementary insurance programme aiming to extend the coverage of insurance by increasing both the rate and the upper limit of reimbursement. In this guideline, social insurers are suggested to reinsure with private insurance companies to improve the coverage, while government will take the lead role in designing and managing the 'Catastrophic medical insurance programme'. In 2014, the 'Catastrophic medical insurance programme' has covered about 400 million people in 28 provinces.[13]

There are two major reasons to initiate the catastrophic medical insurance. First, the affordability of health care services is a concern. The catastrophic medical insurance, which focuses on relieving financial burdens of the patients who are swamped by catastrophic medical expenditure, is going to improve the depth of the insurance coverage by increasing both reimbursement rate as well as the upper limit of the reimbursement. Second, the professional skills of private insurers are complementary to social health insurer.[14] There are large amounts of accumulated surpluses for social insurance. In particular, the accumulated surpluses of Basic urban employee Health Insurance reached over RMB 810 billion in 2013 compared to RMB 127 Billion in 2005.[15] Many local social insurers are financially sufficient, but they have no adequate knowledge/skills to figure out the financial risks when designing health insurance policies for catastrophic health care spending. By reinsuring with private insurance companies, social insurers take advantage of their professional expertise.

While there are some initiatives in governance reform, inefficiency in the governance of hospitals and social health insurance is persistent. For example, in most cities/counties, there are still three different types of social insurance plans managed by two different government agencies: local health bureau and social security bureau. Inefficiency is associated with the fragmented insurance system. It is reported that currently over 100 million Chinese people have joined more than one social health insurance plan and that over RMB 20 billion are subsidized to people who have enrolled with more than one social health insurance plan.[16] There are two types of inefficiency: first, the government subsidizes an enrollee more than once. Second, an enrollee contributes premium for multiple health insurance plans, while he can only be reimbursed by one insurance plan for health care expenditure.

For the newly initiated catastrophic medical insurance, although authority should be allocated to private insurers with better expertise and information about risk management, private insurers instead play a very limited role in managing the insurance. Given that the principle is that government takes the lead role, private insurance companies do not have much discretion about insurance policy design. Private insurers are usually paid with commission fee for managing the fund while the amount of the commission fee is proportional to the premium of health insurance. For example, in Xiamen city, private insurers are paid at most 3% of the premium contributed to the social health insurance, and government will subsidize private insurers to keep the budget balanced should there be any financial losses for the scheme.[17] In some cities such as Hangzhou, it is the social insurer who directly manages the catastrophic medical insurance.[18]

Governance reform for public hospitals is not very effective either. In most cities/counties, public hospitals are still regulated and managed by local health bureau and the authority of regulation and management are not separated. By 2014, only 6 out of 17 national pilot sites for hospital reform have separated their regulation and management authorities.[19] Some cities initiated the regulatory agency for hospitals under the name of 'hospital management bureau' ('Yi Guan Ju'), but this regulatory agency is still part of health bureau (e.g. in Beijing city, hospital management bureau is a subordinate of health bureau[20]). Decisions made by health bureau are not very credible if these decisions conflict with public hospitals' interests since public hospitals are managed by local health bureau. One illustrating example is the number of medical malpractice disputes is increasing by over 20% since 2002.[21] More people now look for a third party 'People's Mediation' ('renmin tiaojie') to sort out the disputes since People's Mediation, which reports to local justice bureau, is independent from health bureau.[22]

Reallocating of authority in a fragmented political structure

The research question for this article is that given the serious concern of affordability, why the authority is still not allocated efficiently in the Chinese health system? The following discussion will show that the persistence of inefficient authority allocation is a result of the difficulties to reallocate authority in the context of Chinese health reform. To change allocation of authority within a firm depends on the decision of the owner who has the property right. The owner is the residual claimer of a firm, and he can decide who have authority for certain risks (Hart 1996).

However, changing *status quo* allocation of authority within a government-owned/controlled organization such as public hospitals and social health insurances is even more complicated. It depends on whether different government departments involved with management or operation of social health insurances and public hospitals can reach an agreement to do so. It also depends on how the coordination among different government departments can be enforced after reaching an agreement. Furthermore, since health care is a 'resource dependent' and 'nonproductive' sector, health reform, compared to reforms in other policy areas, is even more likely to depend on the coordination amongst various government departments (Huang 2013: 136). For example, there are at least 11 ministries outside health sector involved with the health reform in China (i.e. Table 1). The departmental interests for these ministries are much diversified (Hsiao 2007).

As the most influential model to explain Chinese politics, the 'Fragmented Authoritarianism' literature highlights the critical role in policy making and implementation process of the fragmented and decentralized structure of authority. This fragmented structure can be referred as the fragmentation among government departments (i.e. horizontal) or the fragmentation between central and local level governments (i.e. vertical). Policy making in this context may be ineffective since each government department or different levels of government will bargain with one another in defend of their own interests.

Table 1. Ministries involved in the health reform*.

Health sector	Non-health sectors
National Health and Family Planning Commission (including State Administration of Traditional Chinese Medicine)	Ministry of Human Resources and Social Security
China Food and Drug Administration	National Development and Reform Commission
	Ministry of Finance
	Ministry of Civil Affairs
	China Insurance Regulatory Commission
	State Commission for Public Sector Reform
	Ministry of Industry and Information Technology
	Ministry of Education
	State-owned Assets Supervision and Administration Commission
	Ministry of Commerce
	Ministry of Science and Technology

*The list of ministries is compiled from government guideline for health reform in 2013 and 2014. See the links: http://www.gov.cn/zwgk/2013-07/24/content_2454676.htm and http://www.gov.cn/zhengce/content/2014-05/28/content_8832.htm, Accessed 24 November 2014.

But why does this fragmented structure make it so difficult to reallocate the authority? One quick explanation can be that the number of players is large in this fragmented system. With a large number of players, it is more difficult to have collective actions among various departments with diversified interests (Olson 1965). Following this rationale, given diversified departmental interests in the health reform, it is difficult to reform the hospital governance structure since there are 16 ministries involved in the health reform.[23] However, as Liu (2011) reveals in the case of allocating authority for collecting social security contribution, coordination failures are still there when the number of players is relatively small. There are only two government departments who are involved for collecting social security contribution: tax bureau and social security bureau. Although it is more efficient to reallocate the authority to a single agency to collect the social security contribution, it takes more than 15 years to allocate the authority because these two bureaus refuse to compromise (Liu 2011, p. 155).

Institutions supporting horizontal coordination

This article argues that it is the institutional reasons that explain the persistence of inefficient governance structure in Chinese context. According to the literature of new institutional economics, to achieve coordination and sort out the diversified interests among political actors, similar to a transaction in the marketplace, some institutional arrangements are necessary to facilitate the coordination/exchange of interests.

There are two conditions to be fulfilled for these institutional arrangements. First, an institutionalized platform is needed; where exchange of support among political actors can take place credibly. These institutions reduce the uncertainty for political actors by creating a stable structure of exchange (North 1990). Second, there must be some institutions to make the political actors' coordination credible by limiting the discretion of bureaucracy (Moe 1990). These institutions make sure that the bureaucracy will not shirk in the process of implementing policies made by the political actors.

This article uses the US committee system as an example to illustrate the above-mentioned two conditions for the following reasons. First, with very diverse interest in such a large country, political actors in United States have to deal with the exchange of interests and enforcement issues. For example, legislators have heterogeneous interests since they represent interests located within their districts. Committee system therefore is an institution to coordinate these diverse interests. Second, the committee system is well discussed in the literature as an institution to facilitate exchanges of interest among political actors.

The committee system is pivotal in the policymaking process in United States. Niskanen (2001) argues that the committees are powerful enough to dominate in the legislature in the American political system. In the congress, every committee is associated with a particular policy arena, such as commerce, agriculture, banking, and so on, and every committee has monopoly power in its own policy arena (i.e. its jurisdiction) to change the *status quo* (Sobel and Pellillo 2013). There is a seniority system that a committee member can stay in the committee as long as he intends, conditioning on reelection. In addition, a bidding mechanism works in the congress. Once a member leaves the committee, other congressmen can bid for the seat. Since there is an upper limit for the number of committees a congressman can serve, one has to bid for the most valuable committee for his political interest.

Similar to the case that people make exchanges in the marketplace, legislators can exchange support with other legislators in the political market. For example, legislator A can support legislator B's proposal while in exchange for B supporting A's proposal. However, they are not sure whether the exchange can be made since this exchange may be not simultaneous and flow of benefits can be not contemporaneous.

The committee system facilitates the coordination amongst political actors for two reasons. First, the institutional arrangements under the committee system can facilitate the exchange of support among political actors by providing a stable structure of exchange. The bidding system provides an exchange medium for political support so that a legislator has to bid for the most valuable committee for him. In other words, legislators are sorted by their preferences. In addition, the committees possess monopolized agenda setting power since only a committee is entitled to propose policy changes to legislature in its policy area. Furthermore, seniority system implies that a committee member can always have influence over policies as long as he wishes to stay in the committee. On top of that, bidding system, monopolized agenda setting power and seniority system are helpful to enforce the bargaining results since 'the exchange is institutionalized, it need not be renegotiated each new legislative session' (Weingast and Marshall 1988).

Second, some institutional arrangements support the committee system by making the coordination among political actors more credible by limiting the discretion of bureaucracy. While bureaucrats/government agencies have a degree of autonomy, the congress minimizes the bureaucrats' discretion via *ex ante* controls (e.g. administrative procedure) as well as *ex post* controls (e.g. budget review, sunset review) (McCubbins *et al.* 1987). The administrative procedure requires the bureaucracy to publicize their policy aims *ex ante* and budget review rewards and sanctions the bureaucrats *ex post*. These institutions are useful to induce compliance of bureaucrats to meet the requirement of the political actors.

In short, while United States is not the best example for health reform, the committee system in the United States congress illustrates an institutional solution to coordinate political actors with diverse interests. The committee system fulfils two conditions for facilitating the coordination among political actors. First, the committee system provides a stable structure for legislators to exchange support and enforce bargaining results. Second, some institutional arrangements support the committee system by making sure the coordination is credible in limiting the discretion of bureaucrats with various instruments.

'Fragmented Authoritarianism' and reallocating authority

Both conditions for coordination are not fulfilled in the context of Chinese health reform. A stable institution for coordination among political actors is absent and bureaucrats' discretion is significant.

One should note that there is no clear cut difference between political actors and bureaucrats in China. The ministers/directors in a government department, similar to political actors in western countries, have some political agenda to fulfil. However, these officials are also part of bureaucracy who is responsible for the enforcement and implementation of policies. They are subject to performance evaluation system, in which various tasks are defined by the upper level government (Landry 2008).

The role of bureaucrats is critical in China for two reasons. First, the rules of regulation are set by bureaucrats, it is well recorded in the literature that public policy is a product of bureaucratic bargaining in China (Lieberthal and Oksenberg 1988, p. 4). Compared to bureaucrats in Mao-era China, bureaucrats now are even more influential and have incentives to pursue their goals strategically in the process of policy making (Huang 2013, p. 11). Second, bureaucrats have large discretion over the policy implementation in China. Bureaucrats are exempt from political controls of the legislature. Different from many other countries where executive branch is separated from politicians, 'the executive branch has predominated in the formulation and implementation of regulatory laws and policies' in China (Tam and Yang 2005, p. 6).

In this context, the horizontal coordination in Chinese political system is very difficult to realize efficiently for two reasons. First, at the central level, horizontal coordination among government departments is not institutionalized. There is no stable institution equivalent or similar to the committee system in the US congress to exchange interests for coordinating and enforcing the bargaining results. Currently, at the central and local levels, one solution to coordinate different departments is to establish a small leading group or a coordination group ('lingdao xiaozu' or 'xietiao xiaozu'). For the health reform, there are both central and local level (i.e. provincial and below) small leading groups. Group members are stakeholders for policy making and implementation. For example, there were 16 ministries siting in the coordination group at the central level for health reform, which were renamed as the small leading group for health reform in 2008.[24]

However, unlike the committee system in the US congress, this horizontal coordination mechanism (i.e. small leading group) is not very effective for two reasons. First, in a small leading group, preference structure is not stable. A small leading group consists of various ministries, which are subject to frequent personnel changes.[25] For a given ministry, changes of personnel may imply shifts in the structure of exchange, if different ministers have different political agendas. For example, different health ministers may want to reform health system in different directions and they may have different health reform agenda (e.g. there are five health ministers since 2000). In other words, the structure of exchange of support among government departments is not very stable, given the possibility that political actors can be replaced relatively more quickly for various reasons.

Another reason is that the operation of small leading groups is subject to external shocks. The objective of many small leading groups is to fulfil a certain task[26] rather than to coordinate policy changes in general in a policy area. A new small leading group can be initiated if there is a new task to be fulfilled (e.g. the coordination group for health reform was established in 2006 after the State Council planned to have a major reform in health system[27]). A small leading group can be dissolved after the task is fulfilled (e.g. 2008 Beijing Olympics coordination group was established in 2001 and dissolved after the organizing committee of Olympics took over in 2003). The task-oriented character for the small leading groups implies that this horizontal coordination mechanism is far from stable.

Second, at the local level, the performance evaluation system, as an institutional response to the fragmented structure in the vertical direction, has unintended consequences for horizontal coordination among government departments. Given that bureaucrats have large discretion over the policy implementation, as an institution for *ex post* control, the performance evaluation system for government officials is designed to improve the policy effectiveness by motivating bureaucrats to fulfil policy targets set by the upper level government. Appointment, promotion and demotion of local bureaucrats are decided by whether they have fulfilled the upper level government's requirements for various policy targets. It is also observed in the literature that under the performance evaluation system, local officials in China are likely to be promoted on the basis of growth rate of GDP and fiscal revenue (Li and Zhou 2005, Landry 2008, Shih *et al.* 2012) and social policy targets are not as rewarding (Wu *et al.* 2013).

The theory of bureaucratic behaviour recognizes that bureaucrats usually need to accomplish multiple complicated tasks or a single task which can have multiple dimensions to it (Wilson 1989). Bureaucrats are likely to exert more efforts to carry out observable and rewarding tasks for the sake of performance evaluation (Holmstrom and Milgrom 1991). In this case, local government has strong incentives to allocate fiscal resources on local infrastructure to promote economic growth and broaden tax bases rather than on other less rewarding tasks, which may be in conflict with promoting economic growth. Indeed, local government is efficient in coordination with different local bureaus in terms of infrastructure building and attracting investment (Xu 2011).

The performance evaluation system, as an *ex post* control for bureaucrats, has therefore two unintended consequences. First, local officials are lack of incentives to implement governance reform in the health sector. Governance reform, for local government, is a task which is not as observable and rewarding as infrastructure building since governance reform in the health sector may be in conflict with economic development in the short-term. For example, it is observed that a dramatic increase of infrastructure building in public hospitals nationwide in the past several years. In 2008, there were only 394 hospitals with more than 800 beds, while in 2012, there are 1032 public hospitals with more than 800 beds[28] in the country. Governance reform in public hospitals implies a more restrictive regulation over financial decisions, and as a consequence, infrastructure investment in public hospitals may be decreased. In this case, for local officials, the task of governance reform in hospitals contradicts the target of economic growth, and they lack in incentives to enforce the reform, which may put institutional constraints on infrastructure building in public hospitals.

Second, with the performance evaluation system in which officials in local bureaus are evaluated by local government leaders, local bureaus are likely to be accountable for the local government leaders rather than their ministries when implementing the health reform (e.g. local health bureau vs the National Health and Family Planning Commission (former Ministry of Health)), which makes the coordination among government departments at the central level even more complicated. In many other policy areas, it is observed that ministries have problems to enforce policies at the local level. For example, there is a general insufficiency of coordination between the local government and different ministries in revealing budget information for earmarked transfers, even though these transfers are supposed to be earmarked for particular projects (Wu and Niu 2010).

Discussions

Since 2009, there have been many achievements in the recent round of health reform in China. Ongoing reforms on public hospitals and the new initiated catastrophic medical insurance target at improving the affordability of the health care. Nevertheless, governance reform, which is to reallocate authority in public hospitals and social insurance plans, is still a work in progress.

Institutional constraints are the major reasons why the progress of governance reform is slow. First, there is no institutional arrangement to address the horizontal coordination among ministries and bureaus. Second, the performance evaluation system for officials may distort horizontal coordination among government bureaus for some policy initiatives.

Both institutional reasons imply that government departments at the central level are not very effective in making and implementing reform policies. Explanations for slow progresses of governance reform in this article are consistent with the observations in the existing literature. For example, Huang (2013, p. 137) argues that it is the 'health bureaucrats' and 'local officials' rather than government department at the central level who play 'a significant role' in the health reform.

To understand the importance of reallocation of authority for health insurance and public hospitals is also related to two other issues for the reform in the next phase. First, how to design a better system to take advantage of the interaction of market mechanism and the direct government intervention is an increasingly important question. In some cases, delegating the authority to players from private sector is a better option and, in some others, a direct management by government is more desirable.

Second, the allocation of authority becomes an even more important concern regarding the recent initiative about mixed ownership for public hospital reform. 'Mixed ownership' refers to the situation in which institutional investors from either public or private sectors can invest on public enterprise, including public hospitals. It is believed to be a win–win solution for both public and private sectors given that public hospitals have advantage in human resources (i.e. more qualified doctors and nurses), while the private sector has a larger financial capacity to invest in public hospitals.

In April 2014, a public hospital in Hunan province has been selected as a pilot for mixed ownership reform.[29] In this particular case, government holds 51% of the shares of this hospital, while the rest of shares are held by the investors from the private sector. With more and more mixed-owned hospitals, how to reallocate authority among public hospital managers, local health bureau and institutional investors is an issue to be discussed in the next stage.

Policy implications in this context is that future reform initiatives regarding reallocation of authority should take into account the fragmented structure of decision making in Chinese political system. The other option is to establish a stable institutional arrangement for horizontal coordination and reform the performance evaluation system for officials.

Disclosure statement

No potential conflict of interest was reported by the author.

Notes

1. China health statistical yearbook, various years & Statistical Communiqué on Healthcare and Family Planning Development in China 2013,
2. http://web.yyjjb.com:8080/html/2013-01/11/content_183784.htm and http://money.163.com/13/0207/15/8N4C6SMJ00253B0H.html, accessed 8 February 2013.
3. http://china.caixin.com/2013-09-11/100580817.html, accessed 28 July 2014.
4. http://sbs.mof.gov.cn/zhengwuxinxi/zhengcefabu/201405/t20140527_1084649.html, accessed 4 August 2014.
5. For example, a recent document released by Gaoan city of Jiangsu province in 2011 highlights the importance of the balance in the insurance fund but not much was mentioned about the negotiation mechanism to reduce the treatment fee in the hospital. See http://www.jxhrss.gov.cn/view.aspx?TaskNo=008&ID=105554, accessed 4 August 2014.
6. http://finance.sina.com.cn/china/hgjj/20131115/015417327694.shtml Accessed 8 December 2014.
7. China Reform, No. 8, 2013
8. See http://www.bjah.gov.cn/, accessed 8 December 2014.
9. See http://www.shdc.org.cn/, accessed 8 December 2014.
10. http://news.xinhuanet.com/health/2014-05/13/c_1110654371.htm, accessed 4 August 2014.
11. http://news.xinhuanet.com/health/2014-05/13/c_1110654371.htm, accessed 4 August 2014.
12. http://www.mof.gov.cn/zhengwuxinxi/zhengcefabu/201208/t20120831_679663.htm, Accessed 4 August 2014.
13. http://companies.caixin.com/2014-07-09/100701481.html, Accessed 4 August 2014.
14. Sun Zhigang, 'The catastrophic medical insurance as the key point of improving affordability of health care', *Administrative Reform*, 54-7, Dec 2012. Note, Mr. Sun is the director of the health reform office in the State Council.
15. China Human Resources and Social Security yearbook, various years
16. http://economy.caijing.com.cn/20140815/3658675.shtml Accessed 4 August 2014.
17. See Qiu and Huang (2014).
18. Ibid.
19. 14 July 2014. Jiankang news. http://www.jkb.com.cn/management/2014/0714/345844.html Accessed 1 December 2014.
20. http://china.caixin.com/2011-08-15/100291163.html Accessed 4 August 2014.
21. From a recent report in *Southern weekend*, 6 November 2014, Chinese Hospital Management Association estimates the number of medical malpractice has increased by 22.9% annually since 2002. See http://www.infzm.com/content/105341, accessed 18 November 2014.
22. One example of the quick development is Beijing city. The number of cases was increased by 40% between 2011 and 2012. See http://www.bjsf.gov.cn/publish/portal0/tab68/info14149.htm accessed 18 November 2014.
23. http://news.xinhuanet.com/politics/2009-01/24/content_10713287.htm Accessed 4 August 2014.
24. http://www.chinanews.com/jk/kong/news/2008/10-31/1432502.shtml and http://news.xinhuanet.com/fortune/2008-11/14/content_10355517.htm. Accessed 14 November 2014. From a government guideline for the tasks to be achieved for health reform in 2013, there are 13 ministries involved in the tasks for health reform in 2013.
25. http://www.china.com.cn/guoqing/2013-07/10/content_29379767.htm Accessed 26 December 2014
26. See a report from China Youth Daily about task oriented small leading groups, 10 July 2013. http://www.china.com.cn/guoqing/2013-07/10/content_29379767.htm Accessed 4 August 2014.
27. http://www.chinanews.com/jk/ywdt/news/2006/09-18/791660.shtml Accessed 14 November 2014.
28. China health statistical yearbook, various years.
29. http://news.xinhuanet.com/local/2014-04/17/c_1110290117.htm, Accessed 4 August 2014.

References

Bloom, N., *et al.*, 2014. *The new empirical economics of management*. Cambridge, MA: National Bureau of Economic Research, Working paper 20102.

Bolton, P. and Dewatripont, M., 2012. Authority in organizations: a survey. *In*: R. Gibbons and J. Roberts, eds. *The handbook of organizational economics*. Princeton University Press.

Cheng, T.-M., 2013. A pilot project using evidence-based clinical pathways and payment reform in China's rural hospitals shows early success. *Health Affairs*, 32 (5), 963–973. doi:10.1377/hlthaff.2012.0640

Currie, J., Lin, W., and Meng, J., 2014. Addressing antibiotic abuse in China: an experimental audit study. *Journal of Development Economics*, 110, 39–51. doi:10.1016/j.jdeveco.2014.05.006

Currie, J., Lin, W., and Zhang, W., 2011. Patient knowledge and antibiotic abuse: evidence from an audit study in China. *Journal of Health Economics*, 30, 933–949. doi:10.1016/j.jhealeco.2011.05.009

Gibbons, R., Matouschek, N., and Roberts, J., 2012. Decisions in organizations. *In*: R. Gibbons and J. Roberts, eds. *The handbook of organizational economics*. Princeton University Press.

Gilli, M., Li, Y., and Qian, J., 2014. Logrolling under fragmented authoritarianism: theory and evidence from China. *In*: *Presented at the conference 'China's political economy: theory and evidence'*, 6–7 October, San Diego, CA.

Hart, O., 1996. *Firms, contracts and financial structure*. Oxford: Clarendon Press.

Holmstrom, B. and Milgrom, P., 1991. Multitask principal–agent analyses: incentive contracts, asset ownership, and job design. *Journal of Law, Economics, and Organization*, 7 (special issue), 24–52. doi:10.1093/jleo/7.special_issue.24

Hsiao, W.C., 2007. The political economy of Chinese health reform. *Health Economics, Policy and Law*, 2 (3), 241–249. doi:10.1017/S1744133107004197

Huang, Y., 2013. *Governing health in contemporary China*. Abingdon: Routledge.

Kornreich, Y., Vertinsky, I., and Potter, P.B., 2012. Consultation and deliberation in China: the making of China's health-care reform. *The China Journal*, 68, 176–203. doi:10.1086/666583

Laffont, J.J. and Martimort, D., 2009. *The theory of incentives: the principal-agent model*. Princeton University Press.

Landry, P., 2008. *Decentralized authoritarianism in China: the Communist Party's control of local elites in the Post-Mao Era*. Cambridge University Press.

Li, H. and Zhou, L., 2005. Political turnover and economic performance: the incentive role of personnel control in China. *Journal of Public Economics*, 89, 1743–1762. doi:10.1016/j.jpubeco.2004.06.009

Lieberthal, K.G. and Oksenberg, M., 1988. *Policy making in China: leaders, structures, and processes*. Princeton University Press.

Liu, J., 2011. Resources, incentives and sectoral interests: a longitudinal study of the system of collecting social insurance contributions in China. *Social Sciences in China*, 3, 139–156.

Ma, J., *et al.*, 2012. *Research on national balance sheet in China*. Beijing: Social Science Academic Press.

McCubbins, M.D., Noll, R.G., and Weingast, B.R., 1987. Administrative procedures as instruments of political control. *Journal of Law, Economics, & Organization*, 3 (2), 243–277.

Moe, T.M., 1990. Political institutions: the neglected side of the story. *Journal of Law, Economics, & Organization*, 6, 213–253. doi:10.1093/jleo/6.special_issue.213

Niskanen, W.A., 2001. Bureaucracy. *In*: W.F. Shughart II and L. Razzolini, eds. *The Elgar companion to public choice, Cheltenham*. Northampton, MA: Edward Elgar, 258–270.

North, D.C., 1990. Institutions and a transaction-cost theory of exchange. *In*: J. Alt and K. Shepsle, eds. *Perspectives on positive political economy*. Cambridge, MA: Cambridge University Press, 182–194.

Oi, J., 1992. Fiscal reform and the economic foundations of local state corporatism in China. *World Politics*, 45 (1), 99–126. doi:10.2307/2010520

Olson, M., 1965. *The logic of collective action: public goods and the theory of groups*. Cambridge, MA: Harvard University Press.

Qian, J. and Blomqvist, Å., 2014. *Health policy reform in China*. Singapore: World Scientific.

Qiu, Y. and Huang, G., 2014. The mechanism for the Catastrophic medical insurance program: international and China experiences. *Zhongzhou Xuekan*, 1, 61–66.

Ramesh, M., Wu, X., and He, A.J., 2014. Health governance and health care reforms in China. *Health Policy and Planning*, 29, 663–672. doi:10.1093/heapol/czs109

Shih, V., Adolph, C., and Liu, M., 2012. Getting ahead in the communist party: explaining the advancement of central committee members in China. *American Political Science Review*, 106 (1), 166–187. doi:10.1017/S0003055411000566

Sobel, R. and Pellillo, A. 2013. The politics of elections and congressional oversight. *In*: M. Reksulak, L. Razzolini, and W. Shughart II, eds. *The Elgar companion to public choice*. 2nd. Cheltenham: Edward Elgar.

Tam, W. and Yang, D., 2005. Food safety and the development of regulatory institutions in China. *Asian Perspective*, 29 (4), 5–36.

Weingast, B. and Marshall, W.J., 1988. The industrial organization of congress; or why legislatures, like firms, are not organized as markets. *Journal of Political Economy*, 96, 132–163. doi:10.1086/261528

Wilson, J., 1989. *Bureaucracy. What government agencies do and why they do it*. New York, NY: Basic Books.

Wu, J., *et al.*, 2013. Incentives and outcomes: China's environmental policy. No. w18754. Cambridge, MA: National Bureau of Economic Research.

Wu, S. and Niu, M., 2010. Understanding the direction of China's public budget reform. *Wuhan University Journal: Philosophy & Social Sciences*, 6, 836–844.

Xu, C., 2011. The fundamental institutions of China's reforms and development. *Journal of Economic Literature*, 49 (4), 1076–1151. doi:10.1257/jel.49.4.1076

Has China's new health care reform improved efficiency at the provincial level? Evidence from a panel data of 31 Chinese provinces

Shaolong Wu[a], Chunxiao Wang[b] and Guoying Zhang[c]

[a]School of Public Health, Sun Yat-Sen University, Guangzhou, China; [b]School of Government, Sun Yat-Sen University, Guangzhou, China; [c]School of Public Administration, South China Normal University, Guangzhou, China

China's new health care reform commenced in 2009, and since then a huge amount of financial resources has been invested to improve public access to basic medical and public health services. This study used the data envelopment analysis (DEA) Malmquist methodology and TOBIT models to examine the changing trends in total factor productivity (TFP) and the impact of policy on the efficiency of China's health care system at the provincial level between 2003 and 2011. The results reveal that despite the health care reform, the TFP of both medical and public health services declined after 2009. Moreover, there were larger differences across provinces and regions. The health care reform initiated in 2009 has in fact had a significant negative impact on the efficiency of public health services, while its effect on medical services has been insignificant. On the basis of these results, this article explores the implications for future reform strategies in China.

1. Introduction

For low-income countries with a policy goal of providing universal health coverage, maximizing resource utilization efficiency is as important as raising extra funds for health services. Efficiency measures the amount of output in relation to a given level of input. Many previous studies have pointed out that both developed and developing countries waste substantial amounts of funds and resources in their health care systems (WHO 2010). In some countries, reforms have been adopted to improve efficiency and to provide more health promotion, preventive and treatment services to the poor. Apart from cutting costs, efficiency can be improved through increasing the quantity and coverage of health service provision for the same cost or through gaining greater benefits from investment in the health sector. The latter efficiency improvement strategy has been the focus of many developing countries, including China.

From 1949 to 1978, life expectancy in a relatively poor China increased from 40 years to nearly 70 years as a result of establishment and improvement of public delivery systems for food, health services and other health necessities (Anand and Ravallion 1993). At the World Health Organization (WHO) Alma Ata conference in 1978, China was presented as a successful model for solving health care problems in developing countries. It had achieved the goal of health care for all with relatively low investment. However, the efficiency of China's health care system suffered in the process of market transformation (Wang 2004). A WHO report in 2000 ranked China 144th among 191 member countries in terms of overall health system performance. Many Chinese people complain about the difficulty in accessing medical treatments and the cost of these treatments (Hsiao 2007a). Why is the Chinese health care system highly inefficient? Some studies suggest that insufficient government investment and the lack of insurance are among the root causes (Liu *et al.* 1995, Hsiao 2007a).

Since the SARS crisis of 2003, the Chinese government has increased investment in its public health and health care sectors. In 2009, it introduced the *New Health Care System Reform* policy with a budget of 850 billion yuan (about 125 billion USD) for the following 3 years to improve public access to basic medical and public health services. The new funds were mainly invested in subsidizing enrolment in insurance schemes, provision of a public health services, compensation for the loss of medical facilities caused by essential drugs policy implementation, construction of infrastructure, purchase of equipment and training of health human resources. For example, the Chinese government provided a subsidy of 80 yuan in 2009 (rising to 200 yuan in 2011) for each person enrolled in the New Cooperative Medical Scheme or the Urban Resident Basic Medical Insurance scheme. The per capita subsidy for basic public health services provided by the government also increased from 15 yuan in 2009 to 25 yuan in 2011, and the allocation for community health centres and township hospitals was tied to annual performance evaluation. This huge amount of money generated more primary health care facilities, health human resources and equipment in China's health care system.

In addition to increasing investment, the *New Health Care System Reform* policy also aimed to improve the governance structure in five fields: health insurance, essential drugs, primary care, public health and public hospitals. From 2009, the reform tried to expand the coverage of medical insurance, establish an essential drugs system to meet public needs, improve the primary health care system to guarantee the availability of basic medical services, extend basic public health services to both urban and rural residents, and implement the reform of public hospitals. During the period 2009–2011, most of the targets established by the central government were input oriented, covering areas such as finance, enrolment, human resources and infrastructure. Ultimately, it was widely acknowledged that in a very short period of time, the Chinese government had created a huge medical insurance network and invested heavily in medical insurance. About 1.4 trillion yuan (550 billion yuan, about 80 billion USD, over budget) had been spent on the health sector (Yip *et al.* 2012). However, it is not clear whether the substantial input and policy changes have improved the efficiency of health services since 2009. While inadequate input can certainly limit efficiency (Evans *et al.* 2001), increased input does not necessarily lead to improved efficiency.

The WHO's 2010 report identified 10 reasons for inefficiency in health care systems. One of the most important reasons involves payment systems and incentive mechanisms for health service providers. Fee-for-service payment and profit-driven systems motivate providers to induce unnecessary demand, such as tests, treatments and expensive medicines, which maximize their income but do not provide the best health gains for patients. Therefore, the mainstream suggestion for China's health care system reform is to shift the payment method to capitation or diagnosis-related groups (DRGs) and reduce providers' motivation to increase their income through expensive prescriptions and tests. However, China has not completely reformed its payment system for hospitals. On the contrary, it has adopted the direct payment method of 'separation of revenue and expenditure' for primary health care facilities. Currently, neither the fee-for-service nor the direct payment model is conducive to improving the efficiency of the health care system (Hsiao 2007b, WHO 2010). Furthermore, Yip and Hsiao (2008) suggest that if the Chinese government fails to deal with the root causes of rising health care spending in the current irrational and extravagant system, the money invested by the government will simply be captured by service providers as opportunities for higher earnings and profits. As a result, China's new health care reform policy will not necessarily improve the efficiency of health service provision.

Using panel data for Chinese provinces between 2003 and 2011, this study applies a two-stage data envelopment analysis (DEA) and TOBIT modelling to examine the efficiency of the provincial health care system in China and the relationship between efficiency changes and the new health care reform policy. Through the non-parametric DEA method, the study calculates the relative efficiency of the health care system in each province and the dynamic changes in efficiency over time. Then, a constrained TOBIT random effect panel model is used to analyse the factors influencing the efficiency of the health care system at the provincial level and to verify whether the policy dummy variable significantly affects the efficiency scores of the health care system. Finally, the article concludes with a discussion of the implications of its findings for future health care reform in China.

2. Literature review

Many studies have pointed out serious inefficiencies in China's health care system (Eggleston *et al.* 2008). In the process of marketization reform, the Chinese government reduced total health expenditure under fiscal pressure and the new liberal ideology, and public hospitals and other health care facilities then had to rely mainly on fee-for-service income from patients (Liu 2004, Wang 2004). Market failure and insufficient government investment and stewardship allow providers to seek optimum profit, which leads to rapid cost escalation (Hu *et al.* 2008, Tang *et al.* 2008). To estimate changes in productivity and efficiency in China's health care system, some studies have applied the DEA method, which provides a measure of health care system performance compared with the production frontier. The efficiency of the health care system in China and its dynamic changes have been estimated at country, province and hospital level since 2000. The findings indicated that China's health care system was not performing as well as before the reform and that there was great disparity between the regions in terms of health care provision.

On the basis of the three goals of a health system, namely health, responsiveness and financial protection, the WHO's *World Health Report 2000* assessed the health system performance of 191 member countries. China's ranking of 144 in this assessment indicated low efficiency in China's health system. However, the rank, evaluation indicators and methods used in this report were questioned by some media sources and scholars (Navarro 2000). Using the DEA method and panel data for the period 1993–1997, disability-adjusted life expectancy (DALE) as an output indicator of the health system, and total health expenditure per capita and average educational attainment in the adult population as input indicators of the health system, Evans *et al.* (2001) repeatedly measured and ranked the health system performance of 191 WHO member countries. In their study, China was ranked 52–65 in producing DALE in terms of the average efficiency index, higher than its ranking in the World Health Report 2000. They claimed that the finding that China was very efficient was based on case studies. The DEA estimation results indicate that this is no longer the case. Some developing countries, such as Oman, perform better than China.

The DEA method has been used not only to measure and compare the productivity and efficiency of health systems across countries but also to assess the performance of sub-national health care systems. Ng (2008) used the DEA-Malmquist model to assess the efficiency of China's health care system at the provincial level between 2002 and 2005 and found that the amount of both input and output indicators continuously increased, but the health care system nevertheless suffered a decline in productivity. Whether using service indicators or mortality indicators, pure technical inefficiency was the root cause of this inefficiency, which suggested that China's health care system should improve governance performance. In terms of the technical efficiency of the health care system in the provinces of China, there is still room for improvement in coastal regions compared with the inland provinces. However, another provincial-level study found that the relationship between input (funds) and output (human resources, facilities) was DEA efficient (Han and Miao 2010). The efficiency of the health care system has been affected by health financing policy in China. Using provincial-level panel data for the period 2005–2011 and the stochastic frontier approach (SFA) model, Li's research indicated that China's health care reform policies had a great impact on the health care industry and the operation of medical facilities (Li 2014).

Hospitals play a very important role in the provision of health care services. Their productivity and efficiency greatly affect the performance of China's health care system. A study of hospitals in Guangdong province produced very interesting results: the 463 hospitals sampled were quite inefficient but nevertheless productive between 2004 and 2008 (Ng 2011). This seemingly contradictory result mainly originated from pure technical inefficiency each year and technological progress over time. Ng inferred that the inefficiency results were a reflection of revenue-based hospital behaviours: unnecessary care, over-prescription of drugs and the adoption of high-tech treatments. The findings on the productivity and efficiency of hospitals also show regional disparity. By estimating the efficiency of 57 hospitals whose costs were monitored by the Ministry of Health, Sun *et al.* (2012) found that total factor productivity (TFP) was highest among hospitals in western China and that the TFP of hospitals in eastern China was higher than that in central regions.

Previous studies have estimated the efficiency of China's health care system across countries, provinces and hospitals, but few studies have used the DEA method to evaluate the efficiency of this system since the large-scale input resulting from the 2009 reform. Considering the characteristics and complexity of China's health care system, this article divides China's health care system into two subsystems, namely medical services and public health services, and uses the DEA-TOBIT model to estimate the efficiency and the policy effect, respectively.

3. Methodology

3.1. DEA-Malmquist index

The non-parametric DEA method has been widely applied in health policy evaluation. Most studies have adopted DEA models, such as CCR, BBC and the Malmquist index, to estimate the relative efficiency of health service providers. The first two models are usually used to measure the static efficiency of each decision-making unit (DMU) relative to the production frontiers at the time. Under dynamic conditions, when both efficiency value and technology level may change over time, the Malmquist index is used to capture the total effect and decompose different drivers of efficiency and productivity.

Because it used panel data, this study adopted the Malmquist index to estimate changes in TFP and efficiency for each DMU. Following Fare et al., the change of TFP measured by the Malmquist index is specified as follows (Charnes *et al.* 1994):

$$m(y_{t+1}, x_{t+1}, y_t, x_t) = \sqrt{\frac{d_0^t(y_{t+1}, x_{t+1})}{d_0^t(y_t, x_t)} \times \frac{d_0^{t+1}(y_{t+1}, x_{t+1})}{d_0^{t+1}(y_t, x_t)}}$$

The above formula denotes the TFP change of production function point (y_{t+1}, x_{t+1}) relative to point (y_t, x_t), where x denotes input, y denotes output and t indicates year. $d_0^t(y_t, x_t)$ and $d_0^{t+1}(y_{t+1}, x_{t+1})$ represent DEA efficiency scores for period t and period $t + 1$, respectively. $d_0^t(y_{t+1}, x_{t+1})$ represents the ratio of output in period $t + 1$ in reference to the production frontier based on period t at the same input level. Similarly, $d_0^{t+1}(y_t, x_t)$ represents the ratio of output in period t in reference to the production frontier based on period $t + 1$ at the same input level. On the basis of the assumption of non-constant return to scale, TFP change is measured by the product of technical efficiency change and technology change, which can be decomposed further as (pure technical efficiency change × scale efficiency change) × technology change. TFP change measures how TFP in period $t + 1$ has changed in comparison to its value in period t. A value greater than 1 indicates productivity growth either because cost has been reduced or output has been increased or both. A value lower than 1 indicates a deterioration in productivity, and a value equal to 1 indicates that productivity remains constant over time.

Technology change indicates the shift of the production frontier from period t to $t + 1$. Technical efficiency change indicates how a DMU has improved its efficiency level over time. Pure technical efficiency change measures how a DMU's operational efficiency has changed over time. Finally, scale efficiency change measures how a DMU's current scale efficiency has changed over time. A value of technology change, technical efficiency change, pure technical efficiency and scale efficiency change greater than 1 implies an outward shift of the production frontier and an advancement in technology, enhanced technical efficiency, improved operational efficiency and scale efficiency, respectively. Technology improvement is often caused by cost reduction or efficiency enhancement as a result of technical advancement or managerial innovation. A value equal to 1 means no change. A value of pure technical efficiency less than 1 means that the operational efficiency of a DMU has dropped, indicating a need for greater managerial improvement.

3.2. The two-stage method and the TOBIT model

Many controllable and non-controllable factors affect the efficiency of a DMU. However, the DEA method itself does not take into account the influence of non-controllable factors. In order to estimate whether external factors such as the social, economic and political environment affect the efficiency of different DMUs, the limited TOBIT model was used to explore the association between DMUs' efficiency scores (dependent variable) and external factors (independent variables). Because DEA efficiency scores are censored data between 0 and 1, the limited TOBIT model is better than the traditional ordinary least square (OLS) regression.

3.3. Data and variables

3.3.1. Data

This study took a sample of 31 provinces (also cities and autonomous regions, hereinafter referred to as 'provinces'), and each province was treated as one DMU. The panel data of input and output variables for the period 2003–2011 were collected to estimate each province's health system efficiency by calculating their individual DEA output-oriented Malmquist index. Following the SARS outbreak in 2003, China started to increase investment in the health sector. We chose the period 2003–2011 to estimate the DEA efficiency of China's health system on the basis of considerations of policy implementation and data availability. For data comparability, each province's GDP was computed relative to the base year of 2003 using the consumer price index (CPI) to exclude the effect of price fluctuations over time. All data used to produce the indices were obtained from China Statistical Yearbooks (2004–2012) and China Health Statistics Yearbooks (2004–2012).

3.3.2. Input and output variables for the DEA model

The choice of input and output variables is critical for efficiency evaluation. After consulting with experts and reviewing the relevant literature, we took into consideration data availability and the parametric restrictions posed by the analytical model and selected two input variables: the number of health technical employees per thousand population was selected to be the proxy for human resource input, and the quantity of beds in medical and health institutions per thousand population was chosen as the proxy for material resource input. Medical institutions and public health agencies are two interrelated but relatively independent health service organizations in China, and they differ distinctly in terms of their output. For a more comprehensive evaluation of China's health care system, two different sets of output variables were chosen to estimate its productivity and efficiency (please refer to Table 1 for more details).

3.3.3. Independent variables for the TOBIT model

The independent variables used in the TOBIT model were as follows:

(1) *Policy*: The new health care reform policy is the focus variable affecting health system efficiency.
(2) *Density*: Grossman *et al.* (1999) discovered that public sector technical efficiency is related to economies of scale and that public services are more efficient for a higher population density.

Table 1. Variables for the DEA-TOBIT two-stage model.

Model	Input variable	Output variable	External factors
Medical service model	Number of health technical staff per thousand; number of beds in medical and health institutions per thousand population	Bed occupancy rate (%); hospital physicians' daily clinic visits; physicians' daily hospital visits	Health care reform; population density; illiteracy rate; GDP per capita; urbanization level; regional dummies
Public health service model		Newborn visit rate (%); system management rate for children under 3 years old (%); prenatal diagnosis rate (%); postnatal visit rate (%)	

Source: The authors self-made.

(3) *Urbanization*: An important factor affecting the efficiency of the health sector in China is the Chinese urban–rural dual system. As urban and rural health care policies have different content and are implemented by different departments (Tang *et al.* 2008), urbanization is expected to improve the efficiency of the health care system.

(4) *GDP*: It is believed that a higher level of income or wealth and the ability to monitor the government will together improve the efficiency of government expenditure (Migué *et al.* 1974).

(5) *Illiteracy*: It is evident in both domestic and foreign empirical studies that the efficiency of government spending is positively related to the average education level of the local population (De Borger and Kerstens 1996).

(6) *Region*: As geographical differences are an obvious feature of the Chinese context, this study also used regional dummy variables to measure the influences of regional disparities and characteristics on the health system's efficiency.

The above six independent variables were all control variables, and our focus was on the impact of health care reform policy on health service efficiency. The DEA-TOBIT model used in this study was as follows:

$$Efficiency_{it} = \beta_0 + \beta_1 Policy_{it} + \beta_2 Density_{it} + \beta_3 Illiteracy_{it} + \beta_4 GDP_{it}$$
$$+ \beta_5 Urbanization_{it} + \beta_6 D_k + u_i + e_{it}$$

The independent variable *Efficiency* represents the DEA efficiency scores of provincial health services. To account for the effect of health care reform, the independent variable *Policy* takes a value of 0 for the period before adoption and 1 after. Regarding the other independent variables, *Density*, dividing the size of a province's geographical area by its year-end population, signifies the density of population; *Illiteracy*, measured by the illiteracy rate, indicates the educational level of each province; *GDP* is a proxy for income level and is measured by provincial GDP per capita; *Urbanization*, estimated by the share of urban residents in a province's total population, indicates the degree of urbanization; *Region,* divided into three districts, dummy variables *D1* and *D2* respectively represent central and eastern regions (the western region is the reference group) in China. The random variable *u* changes with individual data but is uncorrelated with time and the explanatory variables. The random variable *e* changes independently over time as well as across individual data. The interpretations for the remaining terms are as follows: β_0 is the constant term of the regression equation; β_1–β_6 are the regression coefficients of corresponding independent variables; *i* stands for DMU, which indicates the number of provinces; and *t* signifies the year.

4. Empirical results

4.1. Descriptive statistics

As noted in Table 2, regarding the input of health resources, more governmental investment in the health sector generates a continuous increase in both human resources and bed investment. The number of health technical staff per thousand population and the number of beds in medical and health institutions increased respectively from 3.89 and 2.66 in 2003 to 5.07 and 4.06 in 2011. As regards the output of medical services, the utilization of bed and human resources became more efficient. Bed occupancy rate, hospital physicians'

Table 2. Descriptive statistics for China's provincial health service input and output variables.

Variables	2003 Mean (SE)	2004 Mean (SE)	2005 Mean (SE)	2006 Mean (SE)	2007 Mean (SE)	2008 Mean (SE)	2009 Mean (SE)	2010 Mean (SE)	2011 Mean (SE)
Number of health technical staff per thousand population	3.89 (0.289)	3.92 (0.292)	3.94 (0.293)	4.03 (0.308)	4.13 (0.340)	4.30 (0.357)	4.65 (0.369)	4.85 (0.383)	5.07 (0.394)
Number of beds in medical and health institutions	2.66 (0.189)	2.71 (0.193)	2.76 (0.195)	3.04 (0.217)	3.14 (0.216)	3.36 (0.209)	3.59 (0.207)	3.83 (0.210)	4.06 (0.203)
Bed occupancy rate (%)	64.17 (1.773)	67.27 (1.796)	68.99 (1.638)	71.19 (1.509)	76.52 (1.618)	78.45 (2.169)	83.63 (1.329)	85.57 (1.362)	87.28 (1.257)
Hospital physicians' daily clinic visits	4.81 (0.306)	4.79 (0.300)	5.13 (0.325)	5.26 (0.361)	5.78 (0.356)	6.08 (0.411)	6.25 (0.388)	6.31 (0.421)	6.73 (0.456)
Physicians' daily hospital visits	1.51 (0.0656)	1.51 (0.0516)	1.62 (0.0539)	1.67 (0.0580)	1.95 (0.0642)	2.13 (0.0656)	2.12 (0.0650)	2.24 (0.0691)	2.39 (0.0764)
Newborn visit rate (%)	83.26 (1.820)	83.57 (1.646)	82.74 (1.860)	83.10 (1.885)	84.02 (1.806)	83.09 (2.362)	85.50 (1.928)	88.91 (1.903)	89.97 (1.846)
System management rate for children under 3 years old (%)	72.97 (2.865)	73.21 (2.614)	72.95 (2.655)	73.19 (2.600)	73.84 (2.468)	74.68 (2.584)	75.65 (2.495)	81.02 (2.300)	84.65 (2.009)
Prenatal diagnosis rate (%)	88.33 (1.362)	88.97 (1.231)	88.57 (1.381)	88.53 (1.500)	90.20 (1.417)	89.90 (1.475)	91.64 (1.415)	93.29 (1.321)	92.95 (1.239)
Postnatal visit rate (%)	83.96 (1.929)	84.69 (1.712)	84.35 (1.838)	84.27 (1.835)	85.10 (1.910)	85.63 (1.941)	87.82 (1.799)	89.90 (1.835)	90.06 (1.905)

Source: The authors self-made. Standard deviations are in parenthesis.

daily clinic visits and physicians' daily hospital visits also increased from 64.17, 4.81 and 1.51 in 2003 to 87.28, 6.73 and 2.39 in 2011, respectively. In terms of the outputs of public health services, the proxies for maternal and child care services were generally improved.

4.2. Medical service efficiency

4.2.1. Dynamic change over time

Based on the Malmquist indices, Table 3 shows that TFP change fluctuated and then decreased over the period 2003–2011. The average growth rate of medical services' TFP was 7.5% annually, with technical efficiency, technology change, pure technical efficiency and scale efficiency increasing by 3.1%, 4.3%, 1.7% and 1.4%, respectively. Therefore, the overall growth in medical service efficiency was caused by the combined influence of all the decomposed factors. The changes in pure technical efficiency and technology level imply that since 1999, the operation and management skills of China's medical service institutions have improved while the technology level of medical diagnosis and treatment has dropped.

4.2.2. Dynamic change across provinces

From Table 4, it can be seen that the medical services' TFP changes were greater than 1 for all provinces, indicating that efficiency increased universally during the period 2003–2011. Huge differences were observed among provinces' TFP growth rates. The fastest increase was experienced by Tanjin, with a growth rate of 16.4%, while Xinjiang's TFP growth rate increased by only 0.9%. The decomposition of the Malmquist index reveals that the enhancement of Fujian's and Shandong's TFP value was the fruit of technological advancement, while both provinces suffered from a decline of scale and pure technical efficiency. The improvement of TFP in Xinjiang was due to the fact that its technical efficiency improvement outweighed unfavourable technology change.

Further analysis showed that besides TFP increasing in all 31 provinces (100%), technical efficiency rose in 26 (83.9%), favourable technology advancement took place in 30 (96.8%), pure technical efficiency improvement occurred in 24 (77.4%) and scale efficiency enhancement was observed in 22 (71.0%). Only a few provinces' TFP decomposition factor showed no change or a decrease (please refer to Table 5 for more details).

Table 3. The Malmquist index and its decomposition for China's medical services, 2003–2011.

Year	effch	Techch	Pech	sech	tfpch
2003–2004	1.082	0.941	1.060	1.021	1.018
2004–2005	1.006	1.030	1.000	1.007	1.037
2005–2006	0.987	0.999	1.005	0.982	0.986
2006–2007	1.036	1.035	0.980	1.057	1.072
2007–2008	1.054	1.664	1.055	1.000	1.754
2008–2009	1.057	0.907	1.022	1.034	0.958
2009–2010	1.006	0.958	1.008	0.998	0.963
2010–2011	1.024	0.964	1.010	1.014	0.987
Geometric mean	1.031	1.043	1.017	1.014	1.075

Source: The authors self-made.

Table 4. Malmquist index for medical services and decomposition at the provincial level, 2003–2011.

Provinces	Effch	Techch	pech	sech	tfpch
Anhui	1.015	1.049	1.005	1.010	1.065
Beijing	1.075	1.030	1.036	1.038	1.107
Fujian	0.994	1.037	0.998	0.995	1.030
Gansu	1.030	1.050	1.032	0.998	1.082
Guangdong	1.000	1.012	1.000	1.000	1.012
Guangxi	1.000	1.037	1.000	1.000	1.037
Guizhou	1.000	1.050	1.000	1.000	1.050
Hainan	1.025	1.032	1.028	0.997	1.059
Hebei	1.007	1.055	0.995	1.012	1.062
Henan	1.025	1.051	1.014	1.011	1.078
Heilongjiang	1.058	1.045	1.035	1.022	1.105
Hubei	1.024	1.042	1.015	1.008	1.067
Hunan	1.026	1.048	1.017	1.008	1.075
Jilin	1.055	1.053	1.033	1.021	1.111
Jiangsu	1.033	1.032	1.014	1.019	1.067
Jiangxi	1.019	1.047	1.005	1.014	1.067
Liaoning	1.066	1.057	1.042	1.024	1.127
Neimenggu	1.044	1.043	1.035	1.008	1.088
Ningxia	1.033	1.054	1.021	1.012	1.089
Qinghai	1.022	1.041	1.001	1.020	1.064
Shandong	0.974	1.055	0.983	0.991	1.027
Shanxi	1.026	1.055	1.008	1.017	1.082
Shaanxi	1.052	1.057	1.034	1.018	1.113
Shanghai	1.068	1.030	1.002	1.066	1.100
Sichuan	1.011	1.053	1.016	0.995	1.064
Tianjin	1.130	1.030	1.073	1.053	1.164
Tibet	1.091	1.063	1.057	1.032	1.160
Xinjiang	1.020	0.989	1.005	1.016	1.009
Yunnan	1.028	1.056	1.015	1.013	1.085
Zhejiang	1.021	1.027	1.000	1.021	1.049
Chongqing	1.006	1.042	1.009	0.997	1.048

Source: The authors self-made.

4.2.3. Dynamic change across regions

With regard to the service efficiency of different regions, Table 6 shows that medical services' TFP increased in all regions. The average growth rates of medical services' TFP were respectively 7.8%, 7.3% and 6.5% annually for the western, central and western regions; these figures were mainly the result of gains in technical efficiency and technology change. However, the western region's medical services experienced unfavourable scale efficiency.

4.3. Public health service efficiency

4.3.1. Dynamic change over time

Based on the analysis of the Malmquist index, Table 7 shows that the TFP value of public health services dropped by 8.5% on average annually from 2003 to 2011. Specifically,

Table 5. Average annual dynamic efficiency change in medical services at the provincial level, 2003–2011.

Dynamic efficiency	Number of provinces	Percentage
Increase		
TFP tfpch >1	31	100
Technical efficiency effch >1	26	83.9
Technical change techch >1	30	96.8
Pure technical efficiency pech >1	24	77.4
Scale efficiency sech >1	22	71.0
No change		
TFP tfpch = 1	0	0
Technical efficiency effch = 1	3	9.7
Technical change techch = 1	0	0
Pure technical efficiency pech = 1	4	12.9
Scale efficiency sech = 1	3	9.7
Decrease		
TFP tfpch <1	0	0
Technical efficiency effch <1	2	6.5
Technical change techch <1	1	3.2
Pure technical efficiency pech <1	3	9.7
Scale efficiency sech <1	6	19.4

Source: The authors self-made.

Table 6. The Malmquist index and decomposition for medical services at the regional level, 2003–2011.

Region	effch	techch	Pech	Sech	tfpch
East	1.048	1.028	1.018	1.029	1.078
Central	1.020	1.052	1.006	1.013	1.073
West	1.018	1.046	1.020	0.998	1.065

Source: The authors self-made.

Table 7. The Malmquist index and its decomposition for China's public health services, 2003–2011.

Year	effch	Techch	pech	Sech	tfpch
2003–2004	1.068	0.928	1.018	1.049	0.991
2004–2005	0.984	0.995	0.986	0.998	0.979
2005–2006	0.980	0.990	0.998	0.982	0.970
2006–2007	0.986	0.977	1.005	0.981	0.963
2007–2008	1.009	0.931	0.992	1.017	0.939
2008–2009	1.069	0.883	1.013	1.056	0.944
2009–2010	1.007	0.982	1.010	0.997	0.989
2010–2011	0.971	1.001	1.000	0.971	0.972
Geometric mean	1.009	0.960	1.003	1.006	0.968

Source: The authors self-made.

technical efficiency, pure technical efficiency, and scale efficiency increased by 2.2%, 1.3% and 0.9%, respectively, while technology change fell by 13.3%. TFP scores decreased for all years, mainly as a result of the decline in technology changes.

4.3.2. Dynamic change across provinces

Table 8 suggests that the TFP scores of public health services in all provinces except Yunnan had a value less than 1, implying a decreasing trend in public health services' productivity in most provinces. The improvement in TFP for Yunnan was due to the contribution of both technical efficiency and technology change. The TFP growth rate varied from 0.919 to 1.049 across provinces. The decomposition of the Malmquist index revealed that almost all TFP rates suffered from the undesirable decline in technology change exceeding the improvement in technical efficiency caused by the rise in scale efficiency and pure technical efficiency.

Table 8. Malmquist indices and decomposition for public health services at the provincial level, 2003–2011.

Provinces	effch	Techch	pech	sech	tfpch
Anhui	0.965	0.952	0.972	0.993	0.919
Beijing	1.042	0.947	1.000	1.042	0.986
Fujian	0.993	0.958	0.998	0.995	0.952
Gansu	1.025	0.969	1.015	1.011	0.994
Guangdong	0.993	0.950	0.998	0.995	0.943
Guangxi	1.000	0.960	1.000	1.000	0.960
Guizhou	1.000	0.983	1.000	1.000	0.983
Hainan	1.027	0.942	1.018	1.009	0.967
Hebei	0.999	0.955	1.000	0.999	0.954
Henan	1.002	0.961	1.008	0.994	0.964
Heilongjiang	1.022	0.960	1.004	1.018	0.981
Hubei	1.003	0.961	1.003	1.000	0.964
Jinan	0.982	0.960	0.998	0.985	0.943
Jilin	1.019	0.956	1.005	1.014	0.975
Jiangsu	1.005	0.950	1.003	1.001	0.955
Jiangxi	0.999	0.954	1.000	0.999	0.953
Liaoning	1.025	0.959	0.997	1.028	0.983
Neimenggu	1.009	0.953	1.007	1.002	0.962
Ningxia	1.020	0.963	1.005	1.015	0.982
Qinghai	1.029	0.959	1.005	1.025	0.987
Shandong	0.977	0.952	0.995	0.982	0.931
Shanxi	1.013	0.958	0.997	1.016	0.970
Shaanxi	1.018	0.957	1.002	1.016	0.974
Shanghai	1.022	0.962	1.000	1.022	0.983
Sichuan	1.000	0.968	1.004	0.995	0.968
Tianjin	1.020	0.943	0.999	1.022	0.962
Tibet	1.011	0.964	1.004	1.007	0.975
Xinjiang	1.016	0.976	1.013	1.003	0.992
Yunnan	1.043	1.006	1.036	1.006	1.049
Zhejiang	1.001	0.949	0.998	1.003	0.950
Chongqing	0.988	0.976	1.000	0.988	0.965

Source: The authors self-made.

Table 9. Average annual dynamic efficiency change in public health services at the provincial level, 2003–2011.

Dynamic efficiency	Number of provinces	Percentage
Increase		
TFP tfpch >1	1	3.2
Technical efficiency effch >1	20	64.5
Technical change techch >1	1	3.2
Pure technical efficiency pech >1	15	48.4
Scale efficiency sech >1	18	58.1
No change		
TFP tfpch = 1	0	0
Technical efficiency effch = 1	3	9.7
Technical change techch = 1	0	0
Pure technical efficiency pech = 1	7	22.6
Scale efficiency sech = 1	3	9.7
Decrease		
TFP tfpch <1	30	96.8
Technical efficiency effch <1	8	25.8
Technical change techch <1	30	96.8
Pure technical efficiency pech <1	9	29.0
Scale efficiency sech <1	10	32.3

Source: The authors self-made.

Table 9 further shows that the TFP of public health services increased in one province (3.2%), technical efficiency improved in 20 provinces (64.5%), one province (3.2%) showed an advancement of technology change, and pure technical efficiency and scale efficiency increased in 15 provinces (48.4%) and 18 provinces (58.1%), respectively.

4.3.3. Dynamic change across regions

Table 10 displays the Malmquist index results across regions and shows that the TFPs of public health services for all three regions – eastern, central and western – declined during the period 2003–2011. The biggest drop in efficiency (5.6%) was suffered by the central region, followed by the east (3.2%) and the west (2.1%). Both positive change in technical efficiency and the negative movement of technology progression explain the variances in the efficiency of public health services in the western and eastern regions, while both technical efficiency and technology change decreased in the central region.

Table 10. The Malmquist index and decomposition for public health services at the regional level, 2003–2011.

Region	effch	techch	Pech	Sech	tfpch
East	1.021	0.948	0.999	1.022	0.968
Central	0.989	0.955	0.984	1.004	0.944
West	1.006	0.972	1.007	0.999	0.979

Source: The authors self-made.

Table 11.   Regression results of the DEA-TOBIT panel model.

Independent variables	Medical services model			Public health services model		
	Coef.	SE	$p > |z|$	Coef.	SE	$p > |z|$
Policy	0.029259	0.016878	0.083	−0.020920	0.009264	0.024
Density	0.000137	0.000017	0.001	0.000007	0.000010	0.475
Illiteracy	−0.006410	0.001011	0.001	−0.007820	0.000612	0.001
GDP	−0.702730	0.074219	0.001	−0.184080	0.043914	0.001
Urbanization	0.000001	0.000001	0.376	0.000001	0.000001	0.520
Region						
D1	−0.061340	0.016150	0.001	−0.04868	0.009813	0.001
D2	0.010695	0.018666	0.567	0.012307	0.011105	0.268
Cons	1.116809	0.027212	0.001	1.086138	0.016363	0.001
/sigma u	0.007826	0.011596	0.500	0.000001	0.023977	1.000
/sigma e	0.091284	0.004179	0.001	0.055508	0.002492	0.001
rho	0.007297	0.021585		0.000001	0.000001	
N	248			248		

Source: The authors self-made.

4.4.   Other factors affecting efficiency

The regression analysis in Table 11 suggests that the health care reform dummies had a negative impact on public health service efficiency but a positive effect on medical service efficiency. Specifically, the health care reform policy's adverse impact on public health services was statistically significant at the 5% level ($p = 0.024$). The result of the policy dummies' impact on public health services is contrary to the theoretical expectations. Although the impact of the policy dummies on medical services accords with the theoretical inference, it was not statistically significant at the 5% level ($p = 0.083$). The evidence here suggests that the health care reform not only failed to improve service efficiency but actually hurt it throughout the health care system. Regarding the control variables, the illiteracy rate, GDP scale and regional dummies affected the efficiency of both types of health service at the 1% significance level. The illiteracy rate was proved to have a significant negative influence on both medical and public health services, meaning that a higher educational level helps to improve health service efficiency. This is consistent with the evidence found in the literature that efficiency in both models has a positive correlation with GDP per capita. As regards the regional dummies, the efficiency of both the public health and medical services of the central region was significantly lower than that of the western region ($p = 0.001$). Population density had a significant impact on the efficiency of medical rather than public health services. Surprisingly, urbanization was shown to have a positive but not statistically significant effect on both medical services and public health services, possibly the result of the dominant position of Chinese public health institutions and the implementation of the equalization policy.

Table 11 presents two components of the variance of random items in the random effect regression model, the estimated value and the standard deviation of the individual effect u and the random error item e. The value of rho represents the percentage of total variance explained by the variance of individual effects (i.e. variance across groups). The estimated value of individual effect u was far smaller than that of random error item e, and the value of rho was almost equal to 0 in both models, indicating that the change in efficiency of each province's health services was primarily explained by random disturbances rather than the variance of the individual effects.

5. Discussion

The findings of this study show that the TFP scores of China's health care system (both medical and public health services) decreased from 2009 to 2011, with a greater deterioration seen in the public health sector. The Malmquist index for most regions was continuously less than 1 over the period under study, and the lowest score was found in the central region. The implementation of the new health care system reform in 2009 had no significant influence on medical service efficiency and significantly reduced public health service efficiency.

5.1. Decrease in health care system efficiency

With regard to dynamic change over time, the Malmquist indices of the medical and public health services have dropped since 2009. This might be because China invested heavily in health infrastructure and medical equipment subsequent to the global financial crisis in 2008. The fall in the health care system's Malmquist index after 2003 is mainly attributable to the deterioration of technology change caused by two factors. The first factor is medical equipment. Since the marketization reform, the major part of health care institutions' income has come from fee-for-service payments. Health care organizations are motivated to purchase cutting-edge medical equipment in order to attract patients under competitive market conditions (Hu *et al.* 2008). However, as happened in Britain (Simmons and Marine 1984), the substantial financial investment of the Chinese government discouraged the purchase and use of sophisticated equipment. The second factor is the implementation of the essential drugs policy, which stipulated that only essential drugs could be used by primary health care institutions. This policy restricted primary health care organizations' scope and ability to diagnose and offer medical treatment and particularly hindered the development of medical specialties and skills.

When it comes to dynamic change across provinces, the Malmquist scores for medical services improved faster for some provinces, such as Beijing (10.7%), Shanghai (10.0%), Tianjin (16.4%), Heilongjiang (10.5%), Jilin (11.1%), Liaoning (12.7%), Shaanxi (11.3%) and Tibet (16.0%). Beijing, Shanghai and Tianjin are China's richest metropolises; they have the best and largest hospitals nationwide and rank at the top in terms of excellence of medical treatment (Tang *et al.* 2008). While other provinces have insufficient money to invest in the health sector, these municipalities are able to purchase advanced medical equipment and keep their leading positions in the medical field. These municipalities, especially Beijing, not only possess the best medical equipment in the country, but also the most competent doctors. Apart from training brilliant doctors themselves, these metropolises succeed in attracting the best doctors from other provinces by providing excellent salary packages and working environments. Patients with various incurable diseases nationwide also come to these cities for treatment, which further improves their competency in diagnosis, treatment and management. Even without technical improvement, the development of scale efficiency and management ability can help the Malmquist index exceed 1 in these municipalities. The other provinces in coastal areas are, with the exception of Tibet, similar to these municipalities. Tibet is a special case as its financial revenue comes largely from central government subsidies. Since 2003, the central government has increased investment in Tibet's health care sector, making facilities, equipment, human resources and public health services more accessible. Unlike in medical services, the decrease in scale efficiency and management effectiveness and the deterioration of technology are big concerns for public health services. It is well known that Yunnan is one of the poorest provinces in China, and its Malmquist index is greater than 1, probably because of the very low initial level of its public health services in terms of technology, management and scale.

Regarding dynamic change across different regions, the Malmquist scores of medical and public health services for the central region were lower than for the west despite the fact that the central region is financially better off. This situation may be the result of differences in monetary investment and health service personnel. Local governments' spending on the health sector is funded by central government subsidies and their own fiscal revenue. The western region receives more health funding from the central government, and therefore it is required to raise a relatively lower proportion of the money it needs to fund the health sector from its own fiscal revenue. The central region is required to raise a larger proportion of its health spending with fewer subsidies because of its better economic development. In fact, local governments in both the western and central regions still do not have sufficient fiscal capability and willingness to meet the central government's requirements for health expenditure, causing the western region to obtain more health investment from governments at all levels. In addition, as the central region is closer to the rich eastern region, where health service staff receive a higher income, the loss of talented medical and technical professionals is more serious in the central region than in the west. As a result, the Malmquist score of the central region is lower than that of the west, and the east has the highest Malmquist score.

5.2. Impact of the new health care system reform

It seems contrary to the reformers' original intention and public expectations that the new health care policy has failed to improve the efficiency of both medical and public health services and has even made it worse. As a matter of fact, such situations are not rare in the history of health care reform around the world. As part of the construction of a welfare society, investment in health sectors increased substantially along with fast economic expansion in the West between 1960 and 1980. However, problems of cost escalation and low efficiency arose subsequently. Taking the United States as an example, medical expenditure surged significantly after the adoption of the Medicare and Medicaid policies. According to the estimations presented in the green books published by the House of Representatives, the cost of Medicare doubled every 4 years from 1966 to 1980 (Brody 1971, Hudson 1978). Poor efficiency was not uncommon, and cost control became an important issue (Dresnick and Roth et al. 1979, Galblum and Trieger 1982).

After the implementation of the new health care policy, the various outputs of the medical and public health services actually increased in China; for instance, the average bed occupancy rate of medical services across Chinese provinces rose from 64.17% in 2003 to 87.28% in 2011, an annual growth rate of 3.92%. However, health investment grew even faster. From 2003 to 2011, the number of beds in medical and health institutions increased from 2.66 to 4.60 per thousand population, an annual growth rate of 7.09%. Given the dramatic increase in input and limited improvement in output, it is not surprising to see that efficiency failed to improve and in fact even worsened. As pointed out by Kornai and Eggleston in their discussion on health care reforms in Eastern Europe

(Kornai and Eggleston 2001), the health sector requires time to act upon reforms in order to maximize output potential under increased investment.

Of course, inappropriate methods of payment are one of the main causes of low efficiency in China. From 2003 to 2011, payments to public health service institutions were made directly out of the government's health budget; in the field of medical services, payment by service item was always the main payment method. The payment reforms of the global budget and DRGs lagged. The direct payment method and payment by service item are regarded as detrimental to efficiency improvement, causing health service providers to slack off or induce demand (Hsiao 2007b). In order to control the escalation of health costs and improve efficiency, it is important to explore the reform of payment methods as the next step of health care reform in China.

5.3. Policy implications

The Chinese government began to make a significantly increased investment in health sectors in 2003, and the scale of investment has been unprecedented since the health care reform of 2009. Due to the limitation of fiscal capacity, in the long run, it is unrealistic for the government to continuously increase health investment at different levels (especially the prefecture and county levels). When insufficient government health investment is no longer an issue, the improvement of health system efficiency becomes the focus. This study shows that the efficiency of China's health systems, as estimated by nine key indicators, has decreased since 2009 and that the *New Health Care System Reform* policy caused this deterioration. This suggests that efficiency cannot be improved by increasing government investment alone. In the next stage of health care reform, the government should focus on improving the operational efficiency of the health care system. Efficiency improvement requires a set of sophisticated governance mechanisms. Although this study cannot answer the question of what mechanisms affect health care system efficiency directly, it can provide some suggestions based on the analysis of input and output variables.

First, apart from increasing the quantity of essential investment in health resources, it is crucial to enhance the quality of such investments, especially the quality of health care human resources. Currently, the health care system in China suffers from an insufficient quantity of human resources as well as poor-quality medical and health care personnel. Second, despite increases in the average frequency of doctors' daily clinic visits and hospital days, both are still far below the health service standard in developed countries. The main reason for this is that doctors working in primary care institutions have a light workload whereas big hospitals are overcrowded with patients. Hence, the capability of primary health care providers should be improved so as to attract more patients to visit primary health care facilities. Third, the improvement of public health efficiency and outcomes requires further effort outside the health sector. On the basis of historical experiences in China, both the efforts of health departments and the participation of the general public are essential to improve public health and the system's efficiency (Sidel and Sidel 1977). In addition, the method of payment needs to be changed. The payment mechanism of health expenditure should be changed from payment by service item to a more diverse mechanism including DRGs, global budget and pay for performance. Meanwhile, the allocation of funds should be changed from direct payment to strategic purchase (WHO 2010). Furthermore, different regions should be treated differently according to a health risk adjustment. Since huge disparities exist across regions in China, the design and implementation of health care reform should be differentiated for different regions. Finally, it is important to speed up the technical innovation of China's health care system. If the technology level advances, for instance making full use of modern information network technology, the efficiency of the health care system can be effectively improved.

5.4. Limitations

First, this study used only nine indicators (two input indicators and seven output indicators) to examine the efficiency of the health care system in China. As the inputs and outputs of the health care system are very complicated, any assessment and evaluation can only provide insight into one aspect of the system. Although this study divided the input and output of the health care system into medical and public health services and endeavoured to select as many as nine key performance indicators, it could only give a partial reflection of the efficiency of China's health care system and implied nothing about other factors. Since 2009, the implementation of a basic public health service policy has included nine categories, but only maternal and child care were examined here because of data availability. Planned immunization and chronic disease management, which achieve great results, were not studied. Second, with regard to the effect of health care reform policy on health system efficiency, the TOBIT model applied in this study could only suggest that the decline in efficiency was correlated to the implementation of the *New Health Care System Reform* policy but could not confirm a causal relationship between the two. Studying the causality between health care reform and health system efficiency requires estimation using randomized controlled trials or quasi-experiments, which is beyond the scope of this article. Third, this study examined the impact of health care reform on the efficiency of China's health care system at the macro level but did not look at the influencing mechanisms in detail. To solve this issue, further research should be conducted at the micro level to investigate how health care reform has affected health care system efficiency.

6. Conclusion

This study applied the DEA-TOBIT two-stage model to estimate the efficiency of China's provincial health services in the period 2003–2011 and investigated the effect of health care reform on health service efficiency since 2009. The findings are as follows: (i) the efficiency of both medical and public health services in China declined from 2009 to 2011; (ii) the efficiency of China's health care system varied significantly across regions as well as across provinces, and the eastern region had the highest level of efficiency; (iii) the health care reform initiated in 2009 had a significant negative impact on the efficiency of public health services at the provincial level, while its effect on medical services was negligible. On the basis of the DEA model, the declining efficiency of China's health care system mainly resulted from unfavourable technology change. Further analysis revealed that substantial fiscal investment has discouraged the use of high technology and new medicine.

The impact of health care reform on efficiency since 2009 has generated new challenges that deserve greater attention. The Chinese government has already invested 3 trillion yuan (about 441 billion USD) in health care reform at different levels. In the long run, the growth of public investment is not sustainable and Chinese policy makers need to find ways to improve the efficiency and effectiveness of the health care system.

There is more than one way to improve the efficiency of China's health care system, the most direct and effective being to reform the payment method.

Disclosure statement

No potential conflict of interest was reported by the author(s).

References

Anand, S. and Ravallion, M., 1993. Human development in poor countries: on the role of private incomes and public services. *The Journal of Economic Perspectives*, 7 (1), 133–150. doi:10.1257/jep.7.1.133

Brody, S., 1971. Prepayment of medical services for the aged: an analysis. *The Gerontologist*, 11 (2 Part 1), 152–157. doi:10.1093/geront/11.2_Part_1.152

Charnes, A., *et al.*, 1994. *Data envelopment analysis: theory, methodology and applications*. New York: Springer Science+Business Media.

De Borger, B. and Kerstens, K., 1996. Cost efficiency of Belgian local governments: a comparative analysis of FDH, DEA, and econometric approaches. *Regional Science and Urban Economics*, 26 (2), 145–170. doi:10.1016/0166-0462(95)02127-2

Dresnick, S., *et al.*, 1979. The physician's role in the cost-containment problem. *JAMA*, 241 (15), 1606–1609. doi:10.1001/jama.1979.03290410038021

Eggleston, K., *et al.*, 2008. Health service delivery in China: a literature review. *Health Economics*, 17 (2), 149–165. doi:10.1002/hec.1306

Evans, D., *et al.*, 2001. Comparative efficiency of national health systems: cross national econometric analysis. *BMJ*, 323 (7308), 307–310. doi:10.1136/bmj.323.7308.307

Galblum, T.W. and Trieger, S., 1982. Demonstrations of alternative delivery systems under Medicare and Medicaid. *Health Care Financing Review*, 3 (3), 1–11.

Grossman, P., Mavros, P., and Wassmer, R.W., 1999. Public sector technical inefficiency in large US cities. *Journal of Urban Economics*, 46 (2), 278–299. doi:10.1006/juec.1998.2122

Han, H. and Miao, Y., 2010. An empirical study of the evaluation and influencing factors for local governments' health spending efficiency: based on the DEA-TOBIT analysis of 31 Chinese provinces' panel data. *Finance and Economic Research (in Chinese)*, 36 (5), 4–15.

Hsiao, W.C., 2007a. The political economy of Chinese health reform. *Health Economics, Policy and Law*, 2 (3), 241–249. doi:10.1017/S1744133107004197

Hsiao, W.C., 2007b. Why is a systemic view of health financing necessary? *Health Affairs*, 26 (4), 950–961. doi:10.1377/hlthaff.26.4.950

Hu, S., *et al.*, 2008. Reform of how health care is paid for in China: challenges and opportunities. *The Lancet*, 372 (9652), 1846–1853. doi:10.1016/S0140-6736(08)61368-9

Hudson, R., 1978. The "graying" of the federal budget and its consequences for old-age policy. *The Gerontologist*, 18 (5 Part 1), 428–440. doi:10.1093/geront/18.5_Part_1.428

Kornai, J. and Eggleston, K., 2001. *Welfare, choice and solidarity in transition: reforming the health sector in Eastern Europe*. Cambridge: Cambridge University Press.

Li, X., 2014. Empirical analysis of total factor productivity growth in China's medical service industry: based on the provincial panel data during 2005-2011. *Chinese Health Economics (in Chinese)*, 33 (4), 55–58.

Liu, Y., 2004. Development of the rural health insurance system in China. *Health Policy and Planning*, 19 (3), 159–165. doi:10.1093/heapol/czh019

Liu, Y., *et al.*, 1995. Transformation of China's rural health care financing. *Social Science & Medicine*, 41 (8), 1085–1093. doi:10.1016/0277-9536(95)00428-A

Migué, J., Bélanger, G., and Niskanen, W., 1974. Toward a general theory of managerial discretion. *Public Choice*, 17 (1), 27–47. doi:10.1007/BF01718995

Navarro, V., 2000. Assessment of the world health report 2000. *The Lancet*, 356 (9241), 1598–1601. doi:10.1016/S0140-6736(00)03139-1

Ng, Y., 2008. The productive efficiency of the health care sector of China. *The Review of Regional Studies*, 38 (3), 381–393.

Ng, Y., 2011. The productive efficiency of Chinese hospitals. *China Economic Review*, 22 (3), 428–439. doi:10.1016/j.chieco.2011.06.001

Sidel, V. and Sidel, R., 1977. *A healthy state: an international perspective on the crisis in United States medical care.* New York: Pantheon Books.

Simmons, R. and Marine, S., 1984. The regulation of high cost technology medicine: the case of dialysis and transplantation in the United Kingdom. *Journal of Health and Social Behavior*, 25, 320–334. doi:10.2307/2136428

Sun, Q., *et al.*, 2012. DEA efficiency analysis of Ministry of Health's 57 hospitals. *China's Health Economy (in Chinese)*, 9, 72–74.

Tang, S., *et al.*, 2008. Tackling the challenges to health equity in China. *The Lancet*, 372 (9648), 1493–1501. doi:10.1016/S0140-6736(08)61364-1

Wang, S., 2004. China's health system: from crisis to opportunity. *Yale-China Health Journal*, 3, 5–49.

WHO, 2010. *World health report-health systems financing: the path to universal coverage.* Geneva: World Health Organization Press.

Yip, W., *et al.*, 2012. Early appraisal of China's huge and complex health-care reforms. *The Lancet*, 379 (9818), 833–842. doi:10.1016/S0140-6736(11)61880-1

Yip, W. and Hsiao, W.C., 2008. The Chinese health system at a crossroads. *Health Affairs (Millwood)*, 27 (2), 460–468. doi:10.1377/hlthaff.27.2.460

Inequality in social health insurance programmes in China: A theoretical approach

Sen Tian[a], Qin Zhou[b] and Jay Pan[c]

[a]Research Institute of Economics and Management, Southwestern University of Finance and Economics, Chengdu, China; [b]National School of Development, Peking University, Beijing, China; [c]West China School of Public Health, Sichuan University, Chengdu, China

Equity is one of the goals of China's new round of health care reform. Results from existing empirical studies provide evidence for the existence of highly unequal distribution of insurance benefits under China's current social health insurance programmes. This paper aims to explain inequity in health insurance by connecting the ways through which insurance programmes are financed with benefit distribution. A theoretical approach is employed, and we find that the inconsistency between insurance premiums and expected benefits among different income levels is the main source of inequity in social health insurance programmes. Our results suggest that the design of premium and reimbursement schemes should be aligned with the income level of the insurant.

Introduction

Over the last two decades, providing affordable health care, housing and education services to the people has been the most pressing challenge for public policymakers in China. Among them, health care has been society's major concern, due not only to the urgency of health problems but also to its complexity. Despite several attempts by authorities to reform the system, there are still significant problems for China's health care system, as can be seen in the wide usage of the phrase 'kan bing nan, kan bing gui (getting medical care is expensive and difficult)'.

Before the economic reform in 1978, China's public health care providers were financed directly by all levels of government. After the market-oriented reform began in 1978, China experienced great economic transitions with significant reforms of the fiscal and health care systems. These measures lead to a decrease in government subsidies to the public hospitals (Pan and Liu 2012, Pan et al. 2013). A large portion of the population bear all medical costs by themselves due to the lack of universal health insurance coverage in the country.

To ease the mounting burden of health care expenditures for individuals, since 2003 China has started to build a comprehensive social health insurance system that aims for universal coverage (Yip et al. 2012). Efforts have been made by the Chinese government to ensure the expansion of social health insurance programmes. An insurance net with universal coverage throughout the country has already been created; this net consists of three major health insurance programmes: the Urban Residents' Basic Medical Insurance (URBMI) for urban small business owners, unemployed and retired population; the Urban

Employee's Basic Medical Insurance (UEBMI) for the urban employed; and the New Cooperative Medical Scheme (NCMS) for all rural residents (Qin *et al.* 2014, Pan *et al.* 2014). The advancement of universal coverage is expected to promote financial accessibility to health care.

While financial accessibility has been promoted in recent years, increasing attention has been given to the problem of equity. In health progressivity literature, equity in health care is assessed by the degree of inequality in paying for health care between households of unequal Ability to Pay (ATP) (Van Doorslaer *et al.* 1993). Inequity occurs when individuals with the same illness but different purchasing power end up with different health statuses. The general notion of equity in health financing involves the value judgement of fairness. It works on the presumption that every member of society has the same right to be healthy and that this right should not be contingent upon one's socio-economic status, particularly income level.

However, beyond this general notion, equity can also have special practical meanings in health care financing. For example, individuals who pay the same health insurance premiums, end up receiving less benefit from the health insurance programmes. When this happens to people with high income, it is called 'positive discrimination'; positive discrimination is often considered to be positive because it indicates that the system favours the disadvantage group so that equity of outcome and distributive justice is maintained. However, when discrimination is against the lower-income population, it is generally considered to be inequitable because it aggravates poverty and widens the wealth gap. Therefore, the equity discussed in this paper is not the same as that discussed in health progressivity research. Consequently, our question of interest is 'do low-income individuals get less than they what paid?' rather than 'do low-income individuals get less than others'?

Social health insurance programmes are one of the most important ways of financing health care. In this paper, we focus on a specific type of equity problem caused by a flawed insurance system. Many researchers have found that low-income groups get less benefit from social insurance programmes, especially in developing countries (Culyer *et al.* 1992, Van Doorslaer *et al.* 2000, Wang *et al.* 2005). When the insurance programme is subsidized by the government, it often results in the phenomenon of 'subsidizing the rich prior to the poor' (Wagstaff and Van Doorslaer *et al.* 1992, Van Doorslaer *et al.* 1999, Wagstaff *et al.* 1999).

However, as pointed out by Huang *et al.* (2007), most of the existing studies on insurance only address part of the whole picture of inequity problems; they either ignore the uneven distribution of insurance benefit or overlook the inequality of insurance financing. This study tries to connect both sides of the equation to present a more comprehensive picture of the problem.

The two sides of the insurance equity problem addressed in this paper – how health insurance is financed and the distribution of insurance benefit – will be discussed in one unified framework. A simple insurance market model will show that the inconsistency between insurance premiums and expected benefit resulting from income differences is the main source of inequity in social insurance programmes. We are also surprised to see that in a fair insurance market with flat premium schemes, low-income insurants are in fact forced to subsidize high-income insurants. Data from China's Urban Resident Basic Medical Insurance (URBMI) supports the predication.

In China, two of the three basic social insurance programmes, URBMI and NCMS, use the flat premium design in which every insurant pays the same premium and enjoys the same reimbursement rate for medical costs. Given the fact that both of the programmes are designed with low premiums along with a low reimbursement rate, our prediction is that the low-income insurant will not be able to afford sufficient treatment due to the high co-payment rates. The underutilization of services by low-income participants in the social insurance programme will ultimately result in the phenomenon of 'the poor subsidizing the rich'. When the government starts to subsidize the social health insurance programme, inequity will be manifested as a reversal transfer payment: 'The government subsidizes the rich prior to the poor'.

Based on these findings, we propose a structural index, the 'unfairness index' (UI), to measure the equity level of a given insurance programme. Compared with other equity measurements based on econometric approaches, UI has its roots in consumer utility optimization and is more straightforward for policy recommendation.

The remaining parts of the paper are organized as follows: Section 2 models the equity problem in a simplified insurance market; Section 3 studies the equity of the URMBI programme; and Section 4 concludes with policy recommendations.

The model of inequity in social health insurance programmes

Income elasticity

In this section, we build a theoretical model to show why insurance schemes with flat premiums will generate an unequal distribution of insurance benefit. By flat premium, we mean that every insurant pays the same premium and has the same coinsurance rate. Inequity may also exist in other insurance schemes with variable premiums, but since the fundamental principle behind these schemes is similar, we focus our analysis on a fair insurance scheme with flat premiums.

The distribution of insurance benefit is actually the result of the insured consumers' equilibrium decisions on how many services to consume. Therefore, we need to analyse the income elasticity of health demand before any judgement can be made on inequity.

Income elasticity of medical expenditure plays a key role in consumer demand. There has been extensive research on income elasticity of health service, and the prevailing opinions are divided into two categories: (1) health service is a luxury good as evidenced by macro-level data shows health expenditures increase faster when income grows (Schieber 1990, Gerdtham *et al.* 1992, Getzen and Poullier 1992, Getzen, 2000); (2) health service is a necessity good, as evidenced by micro-level data in which income elasticity is less than one and, in some studies, indistinguishable from zero (Manning *et al.* 1987, Sunshine and Dicker 1987, Wedig 1988, Wagstaff *et al.* 1989).

These two opinions are not exactly contradictory. In the long run, medical technology continues progressing, the same as the national wealth, and there will always be better treatments even if health input keeps increasing. Therefore, from an historical view, greater health expenditure is always positively related to longer average lifespan and higher quality of medical treatment. However, in the short term, where the medical technology frontier is relatively fixed, heavy investment on medical services is not necessarily beneficial for health. In fact, excessive use of drugs and treatments has been proven to be detrimental. This feature of short-term health expenditure is often captured by micro-level data, where options of what treatment to utilize are usually fixed and there exists a point beyond which more spending provides little marginal benefit. The scenario in our discussion on insurance equity problems is closer to the second category because most insurance funds are balanced on a yearly basis.

However, this does not necessarily mean that income elasticity of medical expenditures covered by social health insurance schemes is less than one or close to zero. It is worth noting that though research using US data may find that income elasticity of medical expenditures is very low, these findings are not necessarily replicable in China or in other developing countries because health insurance in the United States covers most of the population and is relatively successful in protecting low-income families from health shocks. But as for low-income patients in developing countries with limited insurance protection or no insurance at all, health expenditures will often be unaffordable; in these situations, we would observe income elasticity greater than one when using this kind of individual-level data (Sunshine and Dicker 1987, Parker and Wong 1997). From the empirical results, it seems that the impact of income on expenditure is more likely to be through budget constraints than health preferences.

In sum, existing literature on income elasticity seems to support the story of budget constraint. In the next subsection, we will build a simple model to illustrate how budget constraints can result in an equity problem in flat premium insurance programmes.

The social insurance market model

As a risk-sharing device, medical insurance protects the wealth of insurants from the risk of catastrophic medical costs. In addition, for low-income patients, medical insurance has access value (Nyman 1999): it helps low-income patients to go beyond budget constraints, so that they can access health services that they would otherwise be unable to afford. Access value also heavily relies on the insurance payment system because it directly influences final affordability for consumers. For example, access value insurance with low premiums and high co-payment rates would be very limited.

In the following model, we will see the impact of budget constraints on medical consumption decisions.

A consumer's utility function is $V(x, h)$, where h represents consumer's health status and x represents the consumption of other goods. When suffering negative health shocks, the consumer needs to find a balance between health care expenditure m, which will directly influence health status h, and consumption of other goods.

Moreover, we assume the utility function satisfies the 'additivity condition' $V(y - m, m) = U(y - m) + H(m)$, where $U(\cdot)$ and $H(\cdot)$ are both increasing concave functions and y indicates the consumer's total wealth. This assumption is common in theoretical studies in health economics, and it essentially requires that expenditures on health care do not have direct influence on other goods' consumption utility and vice versa.

The consumer has to solve the following problem when facing health shocks:

$$\max_{m} V(y - m, m) = U(y - m) + H(m)$$

$$\text{s.t. } m \leq y$$

The first-order condition (FOC) dictates the best medical expenditure m^* should satisfy the following equation:

$$U'(y - m) = H'(m)$$

The FOC means that, in equilibrium, a consumer's marginal benefit of investing in health should equal his/her marginal loss in consumption of other goods. In this brief model, the wealth level y can have two channels through which it influences medical expenditure m^*: (1) when the budget constraint binds: $m > y$; (2) the increase of y will lower the marginal utility of consumption U', encouraging the patient to spend more on health service: $\frac{\partial m^*}{\partial y} = \frac{\frac{\partial m^*}{\partial y}}{\frac{\partial U'}{\partial m^*} + \frac{\partial H'}{\partial m^*}} > 0$, where $\frac{\partial U'}{\partial y}$ measures the changing rate of marginal utility resulted from the increased wealth.

In this paper, we focus our attention on the first channel, where consumers are faced with budget constraints. As to the second channel, we believe the change of marginal utility is negligible in the wealth range that we are interested in. Therefore, we further assume the consumer's utility function $V(y - m, m)$ to be a quasi-linear form:

$$V(y - m, m) = y - m + H(m)$$

where we assume $H'(m) > 0, H''(m) < 0, \lim_{m \to 0} H'(m) \to +\infty, \lim_{m \to +\infty} H''(m) \to 0$, and the marginal utility of consumption is fixed at one in this formation. We believe this will not be a problem since the subject pool in which we are interested are of low- and middle-income levels, and in a general sense, the marginal utility of money will not start to diminish until it reaches extremely high levels.

Henceforth, the new FOC of the consumer's optimal medical spending becomes: $H'(m^*) = 1$. As for those whose wealth lower than m^*, their $m^* = y$.

Now we consider a case in which every consumer is covered by a fair health insurance that grants the insurer the right to buy medical services at a discounted rate c ($0 < c < 1$) at the cost of the prepaid premium π. Every consumer faces the same health risk with a possibility $(1 - P)$ of being ill and P of remaining healthy. When healthy, the marginal benefit of health care consumption for consumers is zero such that no medical service is needed.

When hit by health shock, the patient's maximization problem becomes:

$$\max_m \quad y - \pi - cm + H(m)$$

$$\text{s.t. } cm + \pi \leq y$$

By the FOC, the consumer's optimal medical spending under insurance is: $m' = H'^{-1}(c)$. Since $c < 1$, it is clear that $m^* < m'$ because when facing discounted medical price, consumers will spend more than necessary since the marginal cost is lower. This phenomenon is called 'moral hazard' and results from an insurance system with co-payment rates (Zweifel and Manning 2000).

Now we consider a simple case in which there are only two types of consumers: n_h high-income consumers with income level of y_h and n_l low-income consumers with income level y_l. We further define the two income levels as $y_l < cm' < y_h$. Medical spending decisions of low-income consumers are always face budget constraints, and they have to pay all their remaining wealth for treatments: $y_l - \pi$.

Fair insurance requires that the ex-post expected insurance payment equals the ex-ante insurance premium:

$$(1-p)\left\{(1-c)m'n_h + n_l\frac{1-c}{c}(y_l - \pi)\right\} = (n_l + n_h)\pi$$

For an insurant with high income, optimal medical spending is m', and it does not change with his wealth as long as $y_h > cm'$. As for a low-income consumer, he/she will receive payment from the insurance company $\frac{1-c}{c}(y_l - \pi)$, because his/her spending is $\frac{(y_l-\pi)}{c}$ under the budget constraint.

Therefore, the expression for the premium of fair insurance is:

$$\pi = \frac{(1-c)(1-P)(m'n_h + n_l\frac{y_l}{c})}{n_l + n_h + (1-c)(1-P)\frac{n_l}{c}}$$

This leads us to the following proposition:

Proposition 1: For insured consumers, the medical expenditure of those with high income will not increase with y_h, but the medical expenditure of those with low income will increase with y_l.

With the help of insurance payments, high-income consumers can reach the optimal point of medial expenditure m', but ones with low income will not be able to do so. Under a co-payment system, the benefit provided to the consumer increases with his out-of-pocket expenditure. Sadly, low-income consumers cannot reach the optimal spending point due to budget constraints; even worse, they are exploited by the insurance scheme because of their inability to pay for enough treatment. Therefore, we have:

Proposition 2: Fair insurance is more than 'fair' for high-income consumers and less than 'fair' for low-income consumers.

Proof: High-income consumers can receive a payment $(1-c)m'$ from the insurance company. That is to say, the 'fair' insurance premium for high-income consumers is $(1-c)(1-p)m'$, such that:

$$(1-c)(1-p)m' > \frac{(1-c)(1-P)(n_h + n_l)m'}{n_l + n_h + (1-c)(1-P)\frac{n_l}{c}} > \frac{(1-c)(1-P)(m'n_h + n_l\frac{y_l}{c})}{n_l + n_h + (1-c)(1-P)\frac{n_l}{c}} = \pi$$

It follows that, because the whole insurance pool is balanced, insurance must be less than fair for low-income consumers.

The reasoning behind Proposition 2 is simple: The low-income consumer cannot pay enough for their treatment. In a flat premium insurance programme, those who consume more receive a relatively larger share of benefit, while low-income consumers who cannot afford enough treatment get less. On the other hand, the budget of a fair insurance scheme is balanced on the aggregate level so that the premium is equal to the average of the expected medical expenditure of the whole population. Now, it is clear that low-income consumers receive less than average benefit and every insurant pays the exact same amount of premium. Therefore, Proposition 2 dictates that low-income consumers are subsidizing the high-income group because the extra insurance benefit from utilizing more services in fact comes from the parts of services that the low-income group cannot afford.

The money the low-income group saved is thus transferred to the high-income group to maintain the fiscal balance of the insurance fund. It turns out that this 'fair' insurance is actually unfair for the low-income group, and part of their premium is consumed by the high-income group. This is why 'the poor subsidize the rich' in flat premium insurance schemes.

Unfairness index

Now that we know the basic mechanism behind the inequity of health financing, a convenient way of measuring the level of inequity in the health insurance programme can be constructed.

Equity in fair social insurance programmes means that the expected insurance benefit $(1 - c)(1 - P)m'$ equals the premium π. Since the high-income group enjoys extra benefit that results from the low-income group consuming less, then the amount of this extra benefit will be a good tool to measure the extent of inequity:

$$UI = \left(\frac{(1 - c)(1 - P)m'}{\pi} - 1\right)\frac{n_h}{n_l + n_h} = \frac{n_h(cn_hm' + (1 - p - cp)n_lm')}{(n_l + n_h)(cn_hm' + n_ly_l)}$$

Essentially, UI is the ratio of expected benefit beyond the premium weighted by group size. It has several merits: (1) $0 < UI < 1$, so that it can be used as direct comparison between different insurance programmes; (2) UI has direct economic implication; by multiplying the total volume of insurance fund with UI, we can get the exact amount of money by which 'the poor subsidize the rich.'

Noted that this formulation of UI only stands in the fair insurance market with flat premiums, and the market consists of consumers only from two income levels. For UI to be applied to other insurance markets, the formulation needs to be altered to fit the specific market setting, but essentially it still should be a weighted ratio of extra insurance benefit.

Inequity of social insurance programmes in China

The insurance financing system in China

The premium system design has direct impact on the affordability of insurance. In developed countries like Europe or the United States, social health insurance programmes usually have no-copay or low co-payment rates for insurants. For example, in the US Medicare program, the inpatient coinsurance rate is around 85% (Medicare and Services 2010, Kaiser Family Foundation 2014, Lieberman *et al.* 2014). Discounted medical prices are cheap and easily accessible so that almost all patients are able to utilize a sufficient amount of treatment. Thus, the income elasticity of health expenditures for insurants is typically near zero (Getzen 2000).

In developing countries like China, the prevailing insurance programmes have low premiums and high co-payments (Wagstaff *et al.* 2009). They do not give the insurant sufficient financial support and risk coverage when health shock occurs.

Table 1 represents the actual co-payment ratios for inpatient care for the three major health insurance schemes during 2007–2011 in China, using the nationally representative data from China's Urban Residents' Basic Medical Insurance Household Survey 2007–2011. (This data will be discussed in detail in the next section.) We can see for

Table 1. Actual reimbursement rate of inpatient in China social health insurance schemes (%).

Year	Total	URBMI	UEBMI	NCMS
2007	63.13	32.34	66.10	36.02
2008	56.23	42.03	63.78	23.22
2009	60.24	42.50	64.42	31.11
2010	63.94	44.21	67.93	46.39
2011	67.34	57.47	71.23	54.69

Notes: (1) Date source: China's Urban Residents' Basic Medical Insurance Household Survey 2007–2011. (2) When calculating the average reimbursement rates, extreme values (top 1% and the bottom 5% samples) are eliminated, except for NCMS samples, because of the limited sample size for NCMS patients.

URBMI, the actual out-of-pocket payment of inpatient consumers constitutes around 60% of their total health expenditure during the 2007–2010 period. In NCMS, this ratio is even higher; from 2007 to 2009, NCMS inpatients paid 70% of total medical expenditures on their own.

Additionally, the presence of a deductible system requires that insurants' out-of-pocket expenditures reach a fixed threshold before any medical consumption can be reimbursed. The same deductible amounts to a larger share of low-income patients' medical expenditure, and this means the low-income group has a higher co-payment rate when they are getting less absolute reimbursement. In this way, the deductible system further reduces affordability for low-income patients.

Using the URBMI scheme as an example, in Table 2 the inpatient samples are divided into five groups according to their income level. The significant gap between the reimburse rate of different income groups can be clearly observed. While the out-of-pocket payment rate of the top 20% income group is nearly 60%, this ratio for the bottom 20% reaches as high as 76.8%. Given the fact that the average disposable income of the bottom 20% income group is 2622 RMB, it is very likely that they will be unable to pay the bills for sufficient medical treatment, even with insurance coverage.

Therefore, we can expect that a substantial number of low-income consumers will receive less than necessary treatment in a high co-payment insurance scheme. Provided that health is not negatively correlated with wealth, low-income patients should have at least the same level of medical expenditure so as to maintain their health. The benefit of insurance with co-payments is tied with expenditure levels. As discussed in the previous

Table 2. Inpatient medical expenditure and reimbursement of URBMI*.

	Total	Top 20% income	Second to top 20% income	Middle 20% income	Second to bottom 20% income	Bottom 20% income
Total medical expenditure	**6651** (10,951)	**8054** (13,752)	**7238** (11,509)	**6673** (11,235)	**5559** (7937)	**4948** (7124)
Reimbursement from URBMI	**2261** (5100)	**3233** (7886)	**2746** (4995)	**2105** (4263)	**1555** (2418)	**1147** (1997)
Out-of-pocket payment ratio	0.660	0.599	0.620	0.685	0.720	0.768
Sample size	1606	378	345	335	315	233

Notes: *Data from China's Urban Residents' Basic Medical Insurance Household Survey 2007–2011. All samples who utilized inpatient services are included.

section, those who spend more can get more from the insurance pool, and those who spend less benefit less.

If the government decides to provide a more-than-fair insurance scheme by subsidizing the insurance funding pool or eliminating its deficit, it is possible for every insurant to receive better insurance in the end. However, the inequity problem brought about by flat premium schemes remains unchanged. High-income patients still receive more than low-income patients. It turns out that government financial support for insurance has a reversal transfer payment effect: 'The government subsidizes the rich more than the poor'.

If a social health insurance policymaker only focuses on balancing the insurance budget at the aggregate level, the inequality problem in insurance will be ignored. It is worth noting that the flat premium design is not the fundamental source of insurance inequality. Even if we relax the flat premium assumption, the problem will persist as long as the insurance premium is inconsistent with the expected benefit. The inconsistency between the insurance premium and its expected benefit is the real source of inequality. It is only when social health insurance policies align premiums exactly with expected expenditure of consumers from different incomes level that the inequity problem can be eliminated.

Analysis of Inequity in URBMI

Data from China's Urban Residents' Basic Medical Insurance Household Survey 2007–2011 give us a brief impression of the inequity problems in China's URBMI programme (Pan *et al.* 2014). There are 157,037 observations in total for the five waves (2007–2011) across nine cities in China of data.[1] Table 3 shows the descriptive statistics of the samples.

Recall from Table 2 that the medical expenditure level falls as income decreases. When the sample is divided into five groups according to income level, the inpatient medical expenditure of the lowest income group is 5361 RMB, significantly lower than that of the highest income group at 7936 RMB. After controlling for the impact of health status and demographic variables, we find that the top three groups do not differ from each other in terms of medical expenditure. However, the two groups with the lowest income spend significantly less than the other groups. Furthermore, the lowest-income group spends significantly less than second-to-last group. This may provide evidence of the impact of budget constraints: Those whose income exceeds their constraints did not spend more than necessary, while the low-income groups must spend all of what they have on health services because they do not receive sufficient treatment. Therefore, we observe a significant, positive relationship between health expenditure and income level among low-income groups; this effect fades away for high-income groups.

Furthermore, there is an ethical issue that needs to be discussed. Many factors like initial health status and health behaviour vary among individuals, and variation in these factors could lead to a difference in medical expenditure. But inequity is only considered to be the uneven distribution of benefit brought about by income differences. As one of the most influential public policy tools, social health insurance programmes should be applied in such a way that social justice among different income groups can be maintained, like regressive taxes or transfer payments. Yet the flat premium insurance programmes are actually a series of reversal transfer payments: either the low-income insurant is paying for health services for the high-income group or the government is subsiding high-income groups more than low-income ones.

Table 3. Descriptive statistics of the national household survey of URBMI.

	Whole sample		Bottom 20% income group		Other income level groups	
	Mean	Standard error	Mean	Standard error	Mean	Standard error
Female sample proportion	0.57	0.49	0.57	0.50	0.57	0.49
Age	38.37	23.26	42.61	21.45	37.29	23.58
Marital status (proportion)						
Single	0.38	0.49	0.29	0.45	0.40	0.49
Cohabitation with partner	0.52	0.50	0.54	0.50	0.51	0.50
Divorce	0.10	0.30	0.17	0.38	0.09	0.28
Education level (proportion)						
Elementary or lower	0.40	0.49	0.40	0.500	0.40	0.49
Junior high school	0.29	0.46	0.34	0.47	0.28	0.45
Senior high school	0.24	0.42	0.22	0.42	0.24	0.43
University	0.07	0.26	0.05	0.21	0.08	0.27
Employment status (proportion):						
Unstable employment	0.52	0.50	0.70	0.46	0.47	0.50
Stable employment	0.05	0.21	0.02	0.13	0.05	0.22
Student or children	0.33	0.47	0.22	0.41	0.36	0.48
Retirement	0.11	0.31	0.06	0.24	0.12	0.32
Chronic disease (proportion)	0.21	0.41	0.31	0.46	0.18	0.39
Family size (heads)	3.37	1.26	3.48	1.39	3.35	1.22
Distant to the nearest hospital (hours to travel)	0.21	0.15	0.23	0.17	0.20	0.14
Family income per person (RMB)	9871	10,766	2622	872	11,683	11,326

Notes: Data from China's Urban Residents' Basic Medical Insurance Household Survey 2007–2011. All samples are included.

As shown in Table 2, the deductible system exacerbates the inequity. The deductible rate is different between cities, but overall, it is rather high relative to the average medical expenditure level. The actual reimbursement rate of the highest income group is 40%, while this rate is only 28% for the lowest income group, indicating that the deductible constitutes a large share of low-income patients' expenditures.

Policy recommendations

In the previous sections, we find a considerable gap of medical expenditures between the rich and the poor. It is clear that the problem of inequity exists within social health insurance programmes with flat premiums and the same reimbursement. Low-income insurants who contribute the same premium and acquire the same benefits package end up with less expected benefit.

The social health insurance programme plays an important role in weaving a safety net for people, and the distributional justice should be valued. Drawing from the findings of this study, several policy adjustments with low application costs could be issued to help solve the inequity problem raised by the flat premium and coinsurance rate design.

The first and the most obvious way is to align insurance premiums with income levels while keeping co-payment levels stable and flat. Premiums should correspond with income such that high-income patients should pay higher premiums than low-income patients. Like the UEBMI programme in China, this system would adopt a progressive premium method (income based) with higher income insurants paying higher premiums. The spirit of this inequality-proof premium system design is to match the variation of premium levels exactly to the differences of expected benefit brought by income differences.

The second way to address the problem is to divide the whole insurance programme into many different sub-programmes according to income level. In this scheme, those who have a similar level of wealth would be required to enrol in the same sub-programme, and each sub-programme would be balanced separately. In this way, the income differences would no longer generate any significant gap in expected benefit. Therefore, each sub-programme would be a fair insurance programme, and government subsidies could target certain groups, like the sub-programme for the lowest income population.

The final solution is to lower the co-payment rate for the social health insurance programmes. This measure has been widely applied in most developed countries and some developing countries. The inequity problem resulting from flat premiums and low deductibles can be minimized by decreasing the co-payment rate. If health insurance covers almost all the financial risks resulting from health problems, low-income insurants would no longer be faced with budget constraints. In the United States, the government provides low co-payment insurance programmes like Medicare and Medicaid for the elderly and for low-income individuals, respectively. In this case, not only would the inequity problem be resolved, but the social health insurance programme would play a maximum role in promoting financial accessibility to health care. However, the higher reimbursement rate programme usually requires higher investments by the government, which is restricted by the country's fiscal system and economic development.

However, low co-payment rates may result in problems such as moral hazard (Zweifel and Manning 2000). Since out-of-pocket payments become negligibly compared with the original price, the demand for medical services may be inelastic to price, resulting in over consumption of health care and loss of social welfare. Moral hazard might bring heavy fiscal burden to the health system, especially when the low co-payment programme is subsidized by the government. To prevent this problem, the first priority is to change the incentives of the health care delivery system. If physicians do not have incentive to encourage excessive consumption, they will not 'conspire' with patients for over pre-scription. There are several solutions. In the United States, health service organizations like health maintenance organizations (HMOs) integrate insurance providers and service providers so that service providers will consider the interests of insurance provider when conducting treatments. Another option is the pre-payment design where the insurer can prepay for treatments for the whole insured group to the local service provider with the lowest practicing cost. In this way, hospitals will fully carry the cost of providing treatment so that over prescription can be avoided.

In conclusion, the risk pooling effect and the access value are what make health insurance programmes important and desirable. The first and second workarounds solve the problem of inequality in payment, but they do not change the value of insurance. Low-income insurants who cannot afford sufficient treatments are no better off in the new system. The third solution provides an answer to this problem by lowering the co-payment rate to an affordable level. These solutions eliminate the inequity problem while at the same time promoting risk pooling and access value by insurance programmes.

We nevertheless recognize that this study has a number of limitations. First, further research is needed to assess how to econometrically estimate the UI. Second, the descriptive method applied in data analysis does control for additional factors; other variables affecting both income and health expenditure might have been overlooked. Third, the proposition derived from the model partially relies on the assumption of quasi-linear utility; the condition for general preference form still needs to be specified. Nationally representative data and econometric models should be employed in future research to help empirically estimate the level of equity in China's social health insurance programmes.

Disclosure statement

No potential conflict of interest was reported by the authors.

Funding

We are grateful to the National Natural Science Foundation of China [71303165 and 71303175], the China Postdoctoral Science Foundation [2013M540706, 2014T70863 and 2014M560830], Sichuan University [skqx201401] and China Medical Board [13–167] for their financial support. The authors are responsible for all remaining errors.

Note

1. The nine cities are Jilin, Zibo, Baotou, Xining, Changde, Chendu, Shaoxing, Xiamen and Urumuqi.

References

Culyer, A.J., Van Doorslaer, E., and Wagstaff, A., 1992. Utilisation as a measure of equity by Mooney, Hall, Donaldson and Gerard. *Journal of Health Economics*, 11, 93–98. doi:10.1016/0167-6296(92)90027-X

Gerdtham, U.-G., *et al.*, 1992. An econometric analysis of health care expenditure: A cross-section study of the OECD countries. *Journal of Health Economics*, 11 (1), 63–84. doi:10.1016/0167-6296(92)90025-V

Getzen, T.E., 2000. Health care is an individual necessity and a national luxury: applying multilevel decision models to the analysis of health care expenditures. *Journal of Health Economics*, 19 (2), 259–270. doi:10.1016/S0167-6296(99)00032-6

Getzen, T.E. and Poullier, J.-P., 1992. International health spending forecasts: concepts and evaluation. *Social Science & Medicine*, 34 (9), 1057–1068. doi:10.1016/0277-9536(92)90136-E

Huang, N., *et al.*, 2007. The distribution of net benefits under the National Health Insurance programme in Taiwan. *Health Policy and Planning*, 22, 49–59.

Kaiser Family Foundation, 2014. *State health facts: medicaid benefits* [online]. http://kff.org/state-data/ [Accessed 11 August 2014].

Lieberman, D.A., *et al.*, 2014. Unintended consequences of a medicaid prescription copayment policy. *Medical Care*, 52 (5), 422–427. doi:10.1097/MLR.0000000000000119

Manning, W.G., *et al.*, 1987. Health insurance and the demand for medical care: evidence from a randomized experiment. *The American Economic Review*, 77, 251–277.

Medicare, C.F. and Services, M., 2010. *Medicare hospice benefits*. Baltimore, MD: US Department of Health and Human Services, Centers for Medicare & Medicaid Services.

Nyman, J.A., 1999. The value of health insurance: the access motive. *Journal of Health Economics*, 18 (2), 141–152. doi:10.1016/S0167-6296(98)00049-6

Pan, J., Lei, X.Y., and Liu, G.G., 2014. Health insurance and health status: exploring the causal effect from a policy intervention. *Working Paper.*

Pan, J. and Liu, G.G., 2012. The determinants of Chinese Provincial government health expenditures: evidence from 2002–2006 data. *Health Economics,* 21 (7), 757–777. doi:10.1002/hec.1742

Pan, J., *et al.*, 2013. Disparity and convergence: Chinese Provincial government health expenditures. *PLoS ONE,* 8, e71474. doi:10.1371/journal.pone.0071474

Parker, S. and Wong, R., 1997. Household income and health care expenditures in Mexico. *Health Policy,* 40, 237–255. doi:10.1016/S0168-8510(97)00011-0

Qin, X., Pan, J., and Liu, G.G., 2014. Does participating in health insurance benefit the migrant workers in china? An empirical investigation. *China Economic Review,* 30, 263–278. doi:10.1016/j.chieco.2014.07.009

Schieber, G.J., 1990. Health expenditures in major industrialized countries, 1960-87. *Health Care Financing Review,* 11 (4), 159.

Sunshine, J.H. and Dicker, M., 1987. Total family expenditures for health care: United States, 1980. *National Medical Care Utilization and Expenditure Survey (Series).Series B, Descriptive Report,* 15, 1.

Van Doorslaer, E., *et al.*, 1993. *Equity in the finance and delivery of health care: An international perspective.* New York, NY: Oxford University Press.

Van Doorslaer, E., *et al.*, 1999. Equity in the finance of health care: some further international comparisons. *Journal of Health Economics,* 18, 263–290. doi:10.1016/S0167-6296(98)00044-7

Van Doorslaer, E., *et al.*, 2000. Equity in the delivery of health care in Europe and the US. *Journal of Health Economics,* 19, 553–583. doi:10.1016/S0167-6296(00)00050-3

Wagstaff, A., *et al.*, 2009. Extending health insurance to the rural population: an impact evaluation of china's new cooperative medical scheme. *Journal of Health Economics,* 28 (1), 1–19. doi:10.1016/j.jhealeco.2008.10.007

Wagstaff, A., *et al.*, 1992. Equity in the finance of health care: some international comparisons. *Journal of Health Economics,* 11, 361–387. doi:10.1016/0167-6296(92)90012-P

Wagstaff, A., Van Doorslaer, E., and Paci, P., 1989. Equity in the finance and delivery of health care: some tentative cross-country comparisons. *Oxford Review of Economic Policy,* 5 (1), 89–112. doi:10.1093/oxrep/5.1.89

Wagstaff, A., *et al.*, 1999. The redistributive effect of health care finance in twelve OECD countries. *Journal of Health Economics,* 18, 291–313. doi:10.1016/S0167-6296(98)00043-5

Wang, H., *et al.*, 2005. Community-based health insurance in poor rural China: the distribution of net benefits. *Health Policy and Planning,* 20, 366–374. doi:10.1093/heapol/czi045

Wedig, G.J., 1988. Health status and the demand for health: results on price elasticities. *Journal of Health Economics,* 7 (2), 151–163. doi:10.1016/0167-6296(88)90013-6

Yip, W.C.-M., *et al.*, 2012. Early appraisal of china's huge and complex health-care reforms. *The Lancet,* 379 (9818), 833–842. doi:10.1016/S0140-6736(11)61880-1

Zweifel, P. and Manning, W.G., 2000. Chapter 8 Moral hazard and consumer incentives in health care. *Handbook of Health Economics,* 1, 409–459. doi:10.1016/S1574-0064(00)80167-5

Too little, but not too late? Health reform in rural China and the limits of experimentalism

Kerry Ratigan

Department of Political Science, Amherst College, Amherst, MA, USA

This article provides a preliminary evaluation of health care reforms in rural China, with particular focus on villagers' perceptions of the quality of care and the rural health insurance programme. Based on semi-structured interviews and an original survey of villagers in three provinces, this study suggests that, although recent reforms may have somewhat reduced the out-of-pocket cost of catastrophic illness, rural health systems continue to suffer from serious deficiencies. By examining villagers' perceptions of health care, this article argues that initial conditions and incentive structures interact with local policy styles to impede effective health care reform in rural China.

After three decades of economic reforms and state retrenchment in social policy, grievances related to issues such as health care, food safety and the environment have taken centre stage in China's national dialogue. In response to growing concerns, Beijing has initiated expansive reforms in health care, including increased financial commitments from the central and local levels of government. Improving access and reducing health care costs in rural China have been major goals of the recent reforms, due to the collapse of commune-based health care in the 1980s. The health care reform process has been characterized by experimentalism and decentralization, as local government has been tasked with adapting the implementation of new policies to suit local conditions. While this experimentalist approach was successful in stimulating economic growth, similar tactics have not yielded such positive results in health sector reform. Thus, despite new policies and progressive subsidies earmarked for health care, serious concerns remain.

Why has Beijing's experimentalist approach, which has been extremely successful in promoting economic growth, not produced better outcomes in health care? This article provides a preliminary evaluation of the implementation of health care reforms in rural China, with particular focus on villagers' perceptions of the quality of care and the rural health insurance programme. Based on semi-structured interviews and a survey of villagers in three provinces, my research suggests that, although recent reforms may have made progress in terms of limited goals such as reducing the cost of catastrophic illness, rural health systems continue to suffer from serious deficiencies, including inadequate health infrastructure and rising costs. By examining villagers' perceptions and local variation in health policy implementation, I argue that initial conditions and incentive structures interact with local policy styles to impede effective health care reform in rural China.

The article proceeds as follows. First, I review the research on decentralization and experimentalism in China. Then, I briefly introduce the recent health sector reforms in rural China. Next, I describe the research methods used in the data collection process. Then, using original survey data, I examine villagers' perceptions of local health facilities. Through semi-structured interviews, I identify and specify some of the deficiencies in current rural health systems. Next, I discuss the role of distinct regional governance styles in producing local variation in health care provision and implementation of new policies. Finally, I provide recommendations for further reforms based on villagers' perceptions of current health systems and rural state–society dynamics.

Decentralization, experimentalism, and social policy

Previous research has credited decentralization and experimentalism with catalysing China's dramatic economic growth in the reform period (e.g. Montinola *et al.* 1996, Heilmann 2008). At first glance, a decentralized approach to governance might be unexpected in the context of an authoritarian regime with a strong central state (Remick 2002). The observed subnational variation is less surprising, however, in the context of the personalistic, agency-based nature of Chinese politics. Rather than developing a consistent institutional structure that would constrain policy-making, Chinese leaders have opted for a 'guerrilla' policy style, inherited from the Maoist era (Heilmann and Perry 2011). This approach to policy-making includes an emphasis on experimentation and adaptability, in opposition to the constraints imposed by stable institutions. In terms of division of labour, the central leadership is responsible for grand strategy, while lower levels are charged with implementation. Thus, despite an increasing number of laws and regulations, the Chinese government tends to use the law as a means to an end to achieve certain goals – such as economic development and social acquiescence – rather than formalize a legal system that would fundamentally constrain the state's behaviour.[1] This emphasis on agency, rather than creating enduring institutions, further contributes to subnational variation, as communities are subject to the preferences of their local leaders, with few viable options to hold officials accountable when they engage in illegal or corrupt behaviour. Therefore, despite the centralizing forces of an authoritarian party-state, decentralization and subnational variation constitute fundamental features of Chinese politics.

Reform of the health sector exemplifies the party-state's decentralized, experimentalist style of governance (e.g. Wang 2011). Although experimentalism has been effective in the economic realm, this approach has not yielded such success in health care reform. Why has a policy-making style that was highly successful in stimulating economic growth been much less effective in promoting reform of the health sector? In the following section, I discuss health care reform in rural China, with a focus on the new rural health insurance programme, which demonstrates this style of governance.

Reforming health care in rural China

While the precursors to rural health care reform were initiated by the central government in the late 1990s, reforms were ramped up noticeably beginning in 2003. In particular, the rural health insurance programme, the New Cooperative Medical System (NCMS, *xinxing nongcun hezuo yiliao zhidu*), was rolled out as pilot projects in 2003. The NCMS was intended to address one of the most severe problems in rural health care: the cost of catastrophic illness. Prior to 2003, as a result of economic reforms and state retrenchment from health care, about 90% of rural residents had been left uninsured (Saich 2006, p. 22). Rural residents were often unable to afford medical treatment and catastrophic medical expenditures became a significant cause of poverty, which led to the emergence of two new idioms: 'poverty due to illness' (*yinbingzhipin*)[2] and 'poverty due to catastrophic illness' (*dabingzhipin*) (Wang 2006). One survey from 2003 indicated that 25% of respondents did not visit a doctor because of the prohibitively high cost and the erstwhile Ministry of Health[3] reported in the early 2000s that 22% of the rural poor identified "unmet medical needs" as the cause of their poverty (Saich 2006, p. 22). Many lower-income Chinese were faced with the choice of impoverishment due to medical expenditures or foregoing treatment. In response to this growing problem and consistent with the central government's experimentalist approach to policy-making, the Ministry of Health began to encourage pilot projects of rural health insurance programmes that would establish risk-pooling schemes targeting villagers in particular.

Initiated in 2003 as pilot projects, the NCMS has achieved basic insurance coverage nationwide in rural areas and constitutes a fundamental aspect of health sector reform in rural China. Throughout the early years of the Hu–Wen administration, the Ministry of Health continued to conduct pilot projects and refine the insurance plans for rural and urban residents. As part of this initiative to increase access to health care, the NCMS combines small household contributions with subsidies from the central and local government in a risk-pooling insurance programme. Participation is voluntary, although there have been accusations of coercion from village cadres (Brown *et al.* 2009).

Much of the responsibility for NCMS administration and programme design is explicitly left to local governments, reflecting Beijing's tendency to decentralize policy implementation. As such, reimbursement rates and the specifics of the rural insurance plan tend to vary significantly, sometimes even within the same province.[4] Funding for the NCMS includes transfers from the central government for central and western provinces for each participant, typically constituting about one-third of the NCMS budget. Meanwhile, wealthy, coastal provinces are wholly responsible for funding the NCMS, where the bulk of the funding comes from the provincial and county levels of government. In this way, the programme represents a somewhat progressive attempt at redistribution. The NCMS seems to have increased access to health care. Hospital directors report a large increase in patients and villagers are somewhat satisfied with the new policy, but concerns remain (Interviews with hospital personnel in Hunan and Gansu). Despite shortcomings, the NCMS has been heavily promoted by the central government. Some provinces even include NCMS participation rates as a target on the cadre evaluation system, which is the primary determinant of career advancement for local officials. As a result, NCMS coverage has increased dramatically since the initial pilot projects. By 2010, seven years after the initial pilot projects, the government reported that over 95% of villagers were covered by the programme.

Previous research from health economics has evaluated some aspects of rural health care reform, such as the effectiveness of the NCMS in reducing the burden of out-of-pocket (OOP) payments, particularly with regard to catastrophic illness. For example, Lei and Lin (2009) found that villagers are more likely to seek medical care than prior to the NCMS, but that overall OOP costs for villagers have actually increased as costs of medical care continue to rise and villagers are more likely to seek care with the NCMS in place (including outpatient and preventive care, which are reimbursed at much lower levels by the NCMS). Moreover, while the NCMS may have somewhat reduced expenditures from catastrophic illness, medical expenses continue to be a significant financial burden, suggesting that reimbursement rates will need to rise, particularly for low-income recipients (Sun *et al.* 2009).

While these findings are helpful in identifying some of the accomplishments and shortcomings of current policies thus far, I provide an additional perspective by utilizing original survey data and semi-structured interviews with villagers, local leaders and hospital personnel. These data go beyond previous research to consider villagers' perceptions of health facilities and how local governance factors impact the capacity of the local government to design and implement policy effectively. First, I discuss the nature of villagers' concerns about the NCMS and rural health care. Then, I examine why Beijing's decentralized, experimentalist approach to health care reform has been insufficient to address these concerns.

Data and research methods

There are few ways to elucidate public opinion on social policy and health care in China. Regular public opinion polls on these issues are unavailable and there are few autonomous social organizations that represent popular views. Rural communities are even more isolated and we generally lack systematic information about the perspectives of villagers and village leaders. To better understand villagers' perceptions and expectations of health care provision in China, I utilize both qualitative and quantitative evidence, including semi-structured interviews conducted with county-level officials, hospital personnel and villagers as well as an original survey of over 1000 villagers and village leaders.

I conducted semi-structured interviews in three provinces from 2009 to 2010. The primary goal of these interviews was to make a qualitative assessment: how were the reforms functioning in practice, what challenges had arisen, what was the response and what were the factors that affected implementation across different regions and socio-economic levels. Because the information I was seeking was related to processes and people's experiences with health systems, the method for gathering the data necessitated a flexible and open-ended approach to interviews (Read 2010, Rubin 2012). Therefore, I conducted semi-structured interviews in seven counties in Jiangsu and four counties each in Hunan and Gansu. I purposefully chose three provinces that vary in their levels of economic development, given the importance of economic conditions in social policy implementation. I also selected counties within each province to reflect salient intra-provincial cleavages, including wealth and degree of urbanization. The respondents chosen for interviews were mainly a convenience sample developed through introductions from local scholars. The semi-structured interviews were used to identify major issues in health care facing villagers and provide additional nuance regarding perceptions of health care in rural China. These interviews also informed the design of the survey and the survey instrument. A list of interviews with local officials is provided in Appendix 1; villagers are not listed individually.

To examine broader patterns in health care grievances, I conducted an original survey of over 1000 villagers and village leaders in collaboration with Leah Larson-Rabin (PhD candidate, Department of Political Science, University of Wisconsin–Madison). The survey was administered by enumerators through face-to-face interviews with villagers and village leaders in three provinces: Jiangsu, Hubei and Yunnan (see Figure 1). We chose these provinces to represent some of the socio-economic, demographic and geographic diversity of China.[5] We used a multi-stage, nested sampling design.[6] Because initial conditions for effective health care infrastructure are highly associated with the wealth of the locality, I sought to ensure variation in this characteristic. Within each province, we purposefully chose three municipalities to represent the socio-economic diversity of the provinces.[7] Below the municipalities, localities were chosen in a nested, randomized fashion. Village leaders were a convenience sample in each village and villagers were selected according to a random-walk procedure. The final sample by

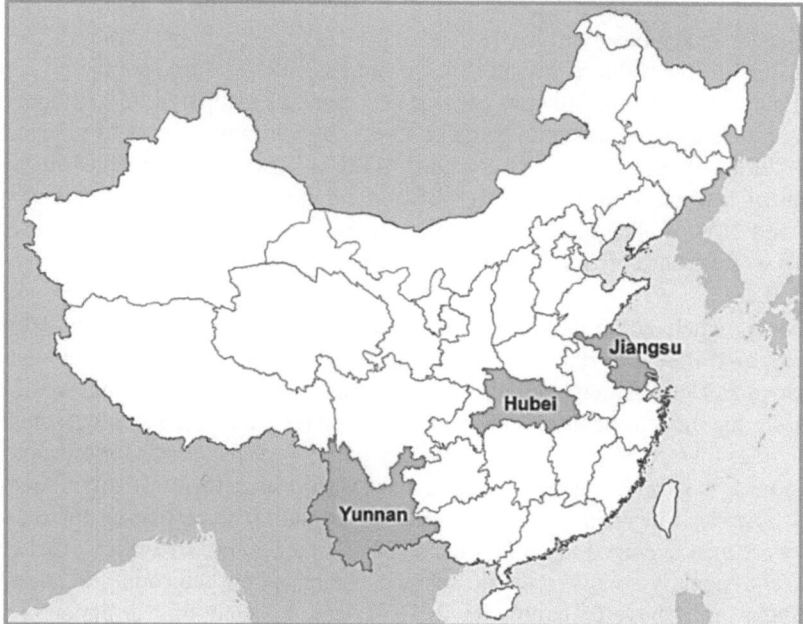

Figure 1.   Map of survey provinces in China.

enumerators comprised three provinces, nine municipalities, 27 counties, 83 townships, 170 villages, 299 village leaders and 801 villagers. The questionnaire included a number of questions about health care use, perceptions and expectations of state health care provision, and demographic information. Overall, our sample of villagers roughly reflects the demographic composition of rural China in terms of gender, ethnic minorities, age, education and Chinese communist party (CCP) membership (see Appendix 2). The survey was conducted in 2012.[8]

Villagers' perceptions of health care

Recent reforms, such as the NCMS, have failed to address underlying deficiencies in rural health systems, particularly in poorer provinces. In general, despite generally progressive policies from the central government, villagers in poorer provinces are more likely to find fault with local health facilities, as evidenced by my survey of villagers. Table 1 summarizes the proportion of villagers in each province that rated as poor or very poor the

Table 1.   Proportion of villagers rating local health facilities as poor or very poor, by province.

	Village clinic (%)	Township hospital (%)	County hospital (%)	Big city hospital (%)
Jiangsu	26	10	3	1
Hubei	29	21	2	2
Yunnan	38	18	0	0

Source: Author's survey of villagers.

quality of local health facilities, including village clinics, township hospitals, county hospitals and big city hospitals.

In Jiangsu, the wealthiest province in the sample, villagers are less likely to rate the village clinic or township hospital as poor or very poor, as compared to their counterparts in Hubei and Yunnan. Villagers in Yunnan are by far the most critical of village clinics, with 38% rating them as poor or very poor. Also, a striking gap emerges in villagers' evaluation of township hospitals: only 10% of villagers in Jiangsu rated them poorly, while 21 and 18% of villagers gave them poor ratings in Hubei and Yunnan, respectively. Villagers' evaluations of local health facilities are presented in greater detail in Appendix 3.

Moreover, when controlling for individual characteristics, villagers in Hubei and Yunnan are more likely to rate local health facilities poorly. Table 2 presents the results of a linear model of villagers' ratings of local health facilities with a number of control variables. In this model, the dependent variable is the respondent's average rating of local health facilities on a scale of 1–5 (5 means very good; 4 means good; 3 means average; 2 means poor; 1 means very poor). Respondents were asked to rate their village clinic, township hospital, township clinics and county hospital. The responses for these local facilities were then averaged to capture the respondent's general perception of local health facilities. The 'poverty county' variable denotes whether or not the county in question had official status as a poverty county in 2011. Locations with this designation receive additional targeted transfers for poverty alleviation efforts. Non-local refers to whether or not the respondent is a migrant to the area. CCP indicates whether or not the respondent is a member of the Chinese communist party. Insurance refers to whether or not the respondent has health insurance (in the vast majority of cases, villagers were participating in the NCMS by 2011). The variable 'contact with village leaders' captures how frequently the respondent interacts with village leaders. The variable 'used health system'

Table 2. Linear model of villagers' evaluations of local health facilities.

Response variable: average rating of local health facilities		
Province	Coeff.	$p > |t|$
Hubei	**−0.291** (0.065)	**0.000**
Yunnan	**−0.283** (0.082)	**0.001**
Control variables		
Poverty county	0.047 (0.062)	0.443
Non-local	−0.053 (0.061)	0.381
Female	**0.132** (0.051)	**0.011**
Age	0.005 (0.010)	0.623
Age^2	0.000 (0.000)	0.986
Income	**0.046** (0.016)	**0.004**
Education	−0.013 (0.028)	0.646
CCP	0.042 (0.089)	0.633
Insurance	0.172 (0.162)	0.289
Contact with village leaders	0.063 (0.049)	0.204
Used health system	**−0.102** (0.056)	**0.069**
Denied reimbursement	**−0.170** (0.074)	**0.022**
Willingness to criticize government	**−0.071** (0.036)	**0.051**
Political participation	**−0.061** (0.029)	**0.037**

Notes: $R^2 = 0.1419$; observations = 604; standard errors in parentheses. Coefficients with a p-value of less than 0.10 are in bold.
Source: Author's survey of villagers.

reflects whether or not the respondent has used a health facility. The variable 'denied reimbursement' denotes whether or not the respondent had been denied reimbursement of medical costs by his/her insurance plan (typically the NCMS). 'Willingness to criticize the government' is captured through the respondent's answer to the following agree/disagree question: 'Everyone should support the government.' (1 means strongly agree; 2 means agree; 3 means disagree, 4 means strongly disagree). 'Political participation' captures the level of participation by the respondent through an aggregate measure of participation in the following activities: political meetings, expressing one's opinion to a higher level political leader, signing a petition and protesting.

Distinct approaches to health policy implementation, coupled with the challenges of implementing health care in an environment where the economy and the health facilities are not as developed as those in Jiangsu, affect villagers' evaluations of local health systems in Hubei and Yunnan. Despite progressive subsidies from the central government, economic factors in less developed regions have caused villagers to continue to have more frequent and dire health-related grievances.

In addition to the clear importance of regional variation, two control variables merit further discussion. Villagers who had used the health system and those who had been denied reimbursement of medical expenditures generally rated their local health facilities more negatively. Certainly, one would expect that a negative experience, such as being denied reimbursement when coverage was expected, would result in a more negative evaluation of health systems. However, merely having used health care facilities is also associated with more negative appraisals of local health facilities. This phenomenon of 'informed disenchantment' – when citizens become more critical of the state after inter- acting with government institutions – has also been observed elsewhere, such as the legal system (Gallagher 2006). This result suggests that local health facilities, particularly in poorer regions, are in dire need of improvement, as villagers who have utilized them tend to be even more critical than those who have not used the system.

These data provide an indication of the general dissatisfaction with health care facilities in rural communities. However, villagers express myriad specific problems with current health care systems that are more readily revealed through semi-structured interviews and focus groups. Using semi-structured interviews with villagers, local leaders and hospital personnel, I identify several specific shortcomings in current rural health policy.

Initial evaluations found that the NCMS has increased the access and utilization of health services by poor, rural residents as well as the volume of care provided, but that out-of-pocket costs and the risk of catastrophic expenditures have not been reduced (You and Kobayashi 2008, Wagstaff *et al.* 2009). For example, my interviews with hospital directors revealed a noticeable increase in patients since the implementation of the NCMS (Interviews JSIH40, JSJH46). One county-level Public Health Bureau official observed that prior to the NCMS, many people would not seek medical attention for 'small illnesses' (*xiaobing*) and, as a result, their illness would become more serious ('big illness', *dabing*). Now, he claimed, people are more likely to go to the doctor for 'small' as well as 'big' illnesses (Interview JSJW44). Although the use of health services has increased, villagers continue to express concerns about the new insurance system.

Perhaps most significantly, despite the NCMS, the high cost of care continues to be a significant problem from the perspective of villagers, particularly for those in poorer provinces, due to several factors. First, most villagers complained of rising prices out- stripping reimbursement rates. According to one villager in Hunan,

'They have to monitor the medical market because after the NCMS some places started to increase prices. In this situation, the NCMS is of no use, [it] does not provide a benefit to villagers and the policy has no significance. So they have to control the costs of production and ensure that hospitals don't charge any inappropriate fees.' (Interview HNDV17, December 2014, 2009)

Some villagers speculate that providers are in fact raising costs because of the NCMS; now that many more people can afford treatment and a significant proportion of the cost is assumed by the state-subsidized NCMS insurance programme, providers see an opportunity to raise prices and increase profits. This option could be particularly tempting for cash-strapped hospitals that have experienced reduced financial support from the state in the reform era.

In addition, many villagers maintain that the current reimbursement rate structure is inadequate. For example, villagers in Hunan, a middle-income province, were more likely to complain that their village health clinic or township hospital was unable to resolve health problems for themselves or their friends or family. As a result, they were forced to travel to the city, typically the provincial capital of Changsha, to receive treatment, where reimbursement percentages for rural insurance are much lower, thereby placing a greater financial burden on the individual (Interviews HNDV17, HNFV53). In a similar vein, villagers in Hunan and Gansu complained that they were not informed by their doctor that certain medications would not be covered by the NCMS, thereby causing further financial stress. Others complained that certain procedures were not covered by the NCMS, resulting in a very small benefit to enrolling in the programme. Approximately half of the villagers interviewed in Hunan cited these issues as a weakness of the NCMS, whereas none of the villagers in Jiangsu raised these problems, even when prompted (Interviews with villagers in all counties). Thus, these targeted policies and the higher reimbursement rates at village and township medical centres in Hunan have not sufficiently addressed the deficiencies in health care infrastructure, such as inadequate treatment facilities and lack of trained personnel in rural areas.

A third concern for villagers is insurance coverage for migrant workers. The NCMS does not always cover migrant workers when they are away from home; coverage and reimbursement rates outside of one's local area vary depending on the specificities of NCMS implementation in one's county of residence. Moreover, when the NCMS does cover out-of-area expenditures, the procedures for reimbursement are often so onerous that they preclude migrants from filing for reimbursement. For example, a migrant worker may be required to file paperwork with the local NCMS office within 30 days of incurring the expense. Many migrants may only return home once a year, at Lunar New Year, thereby preventing timely filing of the necessary paperwork for reimbursement (Interviews with villagers in Hunan). The issue of NCMS coverage for migrant workers was identified as a significant problem early on in the programme's implementation (Brown et al. 2009), but has yet to be resolved in many localities.

In addition to these concerns, there have been scattered reports of corruption related to the NCMS. For example, there have been cases of fictitious patients with fraudulent illnesses filed by providers to extract subsidies from the government ('fake illnesses', *jia bingli*) (Interviews with hospital personnel and media reports in Hunan, 2010). Hospital personnel whom I interviewed in Hunan acknowledged that this was a common problem in the region.

According to villagers and local officials, there are several problems that persist with the NCMS and recent health reforms: reimbursement rates vary significantly across localities; reimbursement rates are lower at higher levels of facilities, which disproportionately affects villagers in poorer localities with less developed health facilities; reimbursement rates are lower for out-of-area facilities, which is a particular problem for migrant workers; drugs that are not on the essential drug list are often excluded from reimbursement, but patients may be unaware of these limitations until they are at the pharmacy counter (Interviews with villagers in Hunan). While recent reforms such as the NCMS have encouraged villagers to seek treatment earlier and, perhaps, have reduced OOP costs in some cases, shortcomings in both NCMS policy and the greater health system prevent recent reforms from addressing serious issues related to quality, access and cost.

Health reform and decentralization

The central government has been extremely successful at incentivizing local government to stimulate dramatic economic growth through a decentralized approach to governance. However, despite a similarly experimentalist process of health reform coupled with progressive subsidies targeting health care in poor provinces, significant challenges remain. Why has the party-state struggled in the social policy realm after such success at promoting economic growth? First, incentives for local officials to promote health care are weak; the cadre evaluation system, by and large, continues to emphasize economic over social targets. In addition, the deficiencies in the health care system are most acute in poorer provinces, despite targeted progressive transfers from the central government. Certainly, economically disadvantaged provinces face greater challenges in terms of both the initial conditions of health care infrastructure as well as general population health due to higher poverty rates. But I propose that incentives and initial conditions are insufficient to explain the deficiencies in health care. Rather, I posit that poorer provinces have developed a style of governance that is not conducive to experimental policy-making. Thus, without explicit direction from Beijing, officials in poorer provinces are not likely to innovate. At best, they tend to implement policies from higher levels pro forma; at worst, directives from above may be perverted due to ineffectual and corrupt local officials. By contrast, wealthier provinces, in general, have been able to find innovative solutions to social policy problems. In this section, I discuss the differences in local governance styles and their implications for the adoption, implementation and, ultimately, effectiveness of social policy with reference to the provinces of Jiangsu and Hunan.

Coastal provinces such as Jiangsu are more economically developed than other provinces. Because these provinces tend to be wealthier than other regions, the central government provides less direct support for social policy and the province is relatively autonomous in terms of social policy provision, both in terms of funding and determining the specifics of policy implementation within broad guidelines established by the central government. In the case of rural health insurance, the central government provides about one-third of the funding for most provinces, with the exception of the wealthy, coastal provinces. Jiangsu, for example, funds the NCMS mainly using provincial and county funds. Wealthier provinces also typically provide more autonomy to municipal and county governments to tailor policy to local conditions. In one city in northern Jiangsu, six rural counties and one urban district decided to standardize their rural health insurance programmes just a few years after pilot projects had begun. They hold monthly meetings within the municipality and have disseminated information among themselves to create a uniform programme (Interviews JSAW01, JSBW07, JSCW10). Notably, this collaborative process was initiated by local actors, rather than the provincial or central governments. By contrast, poorer provinces, such as Hubei and Hunan, have established provincial-level guidelines to standardize the implementation of ostensibly the same rural health insurance programme within the province.

As a result of this relative autonomy in social policy design, wealthy provinces are also more likely to adopt new policies early or to initiate innovative solutions to social policy problems, often resulting in greater within-province variation in social policy provision as compared to poorer provinces. Wealthier provinces are also, therefore, more likely to utilize public–private partnerships in social policy provision. For example, Suzhou in southern Jiangsu is well known for being the first to privatize a hospital (author's fieldwork, 2009). As another example, implementation of rural health insurance in Jiangsu and other coastal regions occurred two to three years prior to implementation in Hunan and other interior regions (author's fieldwork, 2009–2010). Jiangsu has also instituted direct billing for rural health insurance ahead of other provinces (author's fieldwork, 2011). Consistent with State Council regulations (Ministry of Health 2003), wealthier areas are more likely to be chosen for pilot projects and early implementation of new policies (Interviews JSAW01, HNGW30).[9] This approach to pilot project selection reflects a broader strategy for decentralization; wealthier regions are often permitted greater autonomy, while less developed localities are more strictly regulated.[10] Because of these conditions, wealthier provinces such as Jiangsu are more likely to have greater within-province variation in social policy provision, as is the case with reimbursement levels for rural health insurance (author's fieldwork, 2009–2010). The autonomy conferred to wealthier provinces further reinforces a more innovative policy style.

In contrast to wealthier provinces, less-developed provinces such as Hunan are more reliant on central government subsidies for social policy. As a result, these provinces tend to establish regulations to standardize social policy at the provincial level, resulting in a top-down approach to policy-making, less local innovation and less within-province variation. For example, the funding structure for rural health insurance, including per capita contribution levels from the province, county and individual, was standardized at the provincial level in Hunan relatively early on in the policy's implementation, following guidelines set by the central government for the central and western provinces (Hunan Province People's Government Website 2009). Of course, some variation remains and local governments do not immediately comply with provincial regulations, but this effort from the provincial government does tend to reduce within-province variability. Due to the greater involvement of the provincial government, these poorer provinces are generally later adopters of new policy and tend to exhibit less innovation at the local level. For example, rural health insurance was adopted in Hunan several years after adoption in Jiangsu and other coastal provinces.

There are, of course, other exceptions to these tendencies. For example, Shenmu County in Shaanxi province has gained notoriety for using the revenue generated by coal mining to establish an extensive social welfare system for county residents, including universal health care, free education through secondary school,[11] housing subsidies and poverty relief programmes.[12] Although this case could certainly be considered a form of innovation, the governance style in poorer provinces is typically characterized by a top-down, less innovative approach to social policy, in contrast to wealthier provinces.

On the one hand, counties have been given some autonomy to tailor the NCMS and health policy to local conditions, which may, in a virtuous cycle, generate innovation and greater responsiveness to specific local preferences. On the other hand, localities that lack the inclination or the funding to prioritize health policy have lagged farther behind. As health care is tied to one's official place of residence, or *hukou* (residence permit), this creates a 'postcode lottery,' in which residents of poorer localities are even further disadvantaged by less robust social programmes. Thus, the decentralized nature of social policy provision has exacerbated regional inequities in health care provision.

Previous research convincingly argues that the combination of decentralization and experimentalism was a boon to economic growth. However, a similar approach to health reform has not been as effective. Since China has become one of the most unequal countries in the world,[13] it would be far more difficult for local leaders in poor provinces to provide health services comparable to those of wealthy provinces, even given the proper incentives. Moreover, distinct policy styles have emerged that tend to dampen innovation and foster corruption in poorer provinces, thereby exacerbating the deficiencies of the health care system. While this analysis could imply that the path dependence of local policy styles will continue to preclude effective reform, I propose instead that these tendencies could be disrupted with aggressive reform policies, particularly targeting poorer regions. In the current political climate, however, local leaders are unlikely to change their approach to social policy without stronger signals from the central government.

Implications for future reform

Despite clear deficiencies in health systems in rural areas and the importance of health care to villagers, particularly in poorer provinces, we have not observed significant, mass unrest related to health care. Although the state's recent advances in health care have been meagre by objective metrics, these new policies have been subjectively sufficient to ameliorate villagers' grievances, at least for the short term. Therefore, the state has an opportunity to continue to improve rural health systems to keep pace with rising expectations as rural China continues to develop.

Thus far, health reform in rural China has been focused on improving access through cost reduction and some investment in improving basic health systems in villages and urban districts. However, further reforms will need to address rising costs as well as lack of regulation. Additional reforms targeting hospital management and doctor remuneration are currently underway. Despite an increase in government investment in health care, health inequality between urban and rural areas has not abated. Moreover, health care spending is focused on hospital care and urban areas; many rural areas still need investment in basic infrastructure. Without addressing the basic inequities in health care provision, new policies such as the NCMS will have only a minimal effect.

Despite increased state investment in health care, often targeting poorer regions, villagers continue to rate local health facilities poorly. Why have these efforts not achieved greater results? First, local governments continue to prioritize economic growth over social policy programmes. Although the party-state is beginning to include health policy targets in rural cadre evaluation systems in some provinces, these targets are usually soft targets or relatively superficial. For example, participation rates and average reimbursement rates for the rural health insurance programme are now included in cadre evaluations for many localities. Participation rates and other targets are set by higher levels of government and the county aims to reach these targets (Interviews with county officials in Hunan and Gansu). Nonetheless, these targets are typically insufficient incentives to dramatically alter the behaviour of local cadres, as economic growth is still perceived as the top priority (Kung *et al.* 2009; Interviews with county officials in Jiangsu and Hunan). If Beijing is committed to reforming health systems, earnest participation from local officials will be crucial. However, without significant changes in incentive structures for local leaders, beyond simple targets such as NCMS participation rates, it is unlikely that local officials will take social policy implementation as seriously as economic growth.

New incentives for local officials, however necessary, may not be sufficient to ameliorate the abysmal condition of rural health systems in poor provinces, as my research suggests. The central government will also need to consider the ways in which local governance styles interact with existing health systems to impact social policy implementation. For example, villagers' grievances often indicated a lack of profession-alism among practitioners and local health officials, such as a consistent failure to ensure that patients understand their rights and responsibilities, including the cost of various courses of treatment.[14] Strengthening a culture of professional ethics could also address corruption in the health system, such as the problem of 'fake illnesses,' as identified by hospital personnel in Hunan. Reforming rural health systems will require a multi-pronged approach that improves inadequate health infrastructure at the village level, adjusts incentives for local officials and addresses local governance styles. The central govern-ment created the conditions for local leaders to foster unprecedented economic growth in the reform period; it is time for a similar revolution in health and social policy.

Acknowledgements
The author thanks Melanie Manion, Edward Friedman, Christina Ewig and the participants in the Chinese Politics Workshop at the University of Wisconsin–Madison for their comments throughout this research project.

Disclosure statement
No potential conflict of interest was reported by the author.

Funding
The author gratefully acknowledges research support provided by the National Science Foundation Doctoral Dissertation Improvement Grant programme, the Foreign Language and Area Studies Programme of the US Department of Education, the Department of Political Science of the University of Wisconsin–Madison, and writing support from the Chiang Ching-kuo Foundation.

Notes
1. This phenomenon has been described as 'rule by law,' in contrast to the 'rule of law' in democratic systems (Lubman 1999; for a discussion of 'rule by law' in authoritarian regimes beyond China, see Ginsburg and Moustafa 2008).
2. All translations from Chinese are my own.
3. In 2013, the Ministry of Health merged with the National Population and Family Planning Commission and the State Administration of Traditional Chinese Medicine to form the National Health and Family Planning Commission.
4. Since this research was conducted, there have been central government initiatives to standar-dize some aspects of the NCMS, but the primary grievances of villagers as described in this research persist.
5. Jiangsu is the wealthiest, Hubei is middle-income and Yunnan is the poorest and most agrarian in the sample. As a measure of wealth, we used the most recent statistics available for the municipality's gross regional product per capita; these are published by the provincial govern-ment in statistical yearbooks. Jiangsu is located in the littoral region, while Hubei is in central China, and Yunnan is in south-western China (see Figure 1). Jiangsu and Hubei do not have significant populations of ethnic minorities, whereas Yunnan has a large, but varied, ethnic minority population.

6. Publicly available lists of counties and townships were reliable, but additional information that would have been required for a stratified sample of villages was not reliably and consistently available in all provinces. Therefore, we elected to select counties, townships and villages within each municipality randomly.

7. Municipalities, also sometimes translated as prefectures or prefecture cities (*dijishi*), constitute an administrative unit one level below the province that is relatively large. Each province in the sample has between 13 and 16 municipalities.

8. For additional information about the data collection process, please contact the author.

9. Of course, selecting favourable conditions for pilot projects is probably not a wise approach to testing the viability of a new policy, but this issue is beyond the scope of this article.

10. For one explanation of why wealthier provinces are afforded greater autonomy, see Sheng (2010).

11. Typically, nine years of compulsory education, beginning at age six, are virtually free in public schools. Public secondary schools, however, increasingly charge various operating fees that can be a significant burden on lower income families.

12. The county has received some media coverage from the state media for its efforts ('Public welfare programs in Shenmu County, Shaanxi Province,' 2009).

13. Official estimates placed the Gini coefficient at around 0.47 in 2012 (Yao and Wang 2013), but others speculate that it could be much higher.

14. The current practice of medicine suffers from generations of Chinese physicians whose professional careers have been contingent on demonstrating loyalty to the state and communist ideology, in lieu of professional ethics (Lim *et al.* 2004). For more on the need for the professionalization of physicians, see Cao (2011).

References

Brown, P.H., De Brauw, A., and Du, Y., 2009. Understanding variation in the design of China's new co-operative medical system. *The China Quarterly*, 198, 304–329. doi:10.1017/S0305741009000320.

Cao, X., 2011. The Chinese medical doctor association: a new industrial relations actor in China's health services? *Related Industrial*, 66, 74–97.

Gallagher, M.E., 2006. Mobilizing the law in China: "informed disenchantment" and the development of legal consciousness. *Law Social Reviews*, 40, 783–816. doi:10.1111/j.1540-5893.2006.00281.x.

Ginsburg, T. and Moustafa, T., 2008. *Rule by law: the politics of courts in authoritarian regimes.* New York: Cambridge University Press.

Heilmann, S., 2008. Policy experimentation in China's economic rise. *Studies Comparative International Developments*, 43, 1–26. doi:10.1007/s12116-007-9014-4.

Heilmann, S. and Perry, E.J., 2011. *Mao's invisible hand: the political foundations of adaptive governance in China.* Cambridge, MA: Harvard University Asia Center: Distributed by Harvard University Press.

Hunan Province People's Government Website, 2009. *Hunan xinnonghe buchang biaozhun jinyibu tigao (Hunan NCMS subsidy standards take a step further, raised)* [online]. Available from: http://www.longhui.gov.cn/Info.aspx?ModelId=1&Id=25337 [Accessed 4 February 2015].

Kung, J., Cai, Y., and Sun, X., 2009. Rural cadres and governance in China: incentive, institution and accountability. *China Journal*, 62, 61–77.

Lei, X. and Lin, W., 2009. The new cooperative medical scheme in rural China: does more coverage mean more service and better health? *Health Economics*, 18, S25–S46. doi:10.1002/hec.1501.

Lim, M.-K., *et al.*, 2004. Public perceptions of private health care in socialist China. *Health Affairs (Millwood)*, 23, 222–234. doi:10.1377/hlthaff.23.6.222.

Lubman, S.B., 1999. *Bird in a cage: legal reform in China after Mao.* Stanford, CA: Stanford University Press.

Ministry of Health, 2003. Notification of the Opinion of the State Council General Office published by the Health Bureau and other Departments Related to Establishing the New Cooperative Medical System CLI.2.45115.

Montinola, G., Qian, Y., and Weingast, B.R., 1996. Federalism, Chinese style: the political basis for economic success in China. *World Politics*, 48, 50–81. doi:10.1353/wp.1995.0003.

Public welfare programs in Shenmu County, Shaanxi Province, 2009. *Xinhua News Agency* [online]. Available from: http://www.china.org.cn/photos/2009-12/27/content_19138418.htm [Accessed 4 February 2015].

Read, B.L., 2010. More than an interview, less than sedaka: studying subtle and hidden politics with site-intensive methods. *In*: A. Carlson, *et al.*, eds. *Contemporary Chinese politics: new sources, methods, and field strategies*. New York: Cambridge University Press, 145–161.

Remick, E., 2002. The significance of variation in local states: the case of twentieth-century China. *Comparative Polit*, 34, 399–418. doi:10.2307/4146945.

Rubin, H.J., 2012. *Qualitative interviewing: the art of hearing data*. Thousand Oaks, CA: SAGE.

Saich, T., 2006. Social policy development in the era of economic reform. *In*: J. Kaufman, A. Kleinman, and T. Saich, eds. *AIDS and social policy in China*. Cambridge, MA: Harvard University Asia Center, 15–46.

Sheng, Y., 2010. *Economic openness and territorial politics in China*. New York: Cambridge University Press.

Sun, X., *et al.*, 2009. Catastrophic medical payment and financial protection in rural China: evidence from the new cooperative medical scheme in Shandong province. *Health Economics*, 18, 103–119. doi:10.1002/hec.1346.

Wagstaff, A., *et al.*, 2009. Extending health insurance to the rural population: an impact evaluation of China's new cooperative medical scheme. *Journal of Health Economics*, 28, 1–19. doi:10.1016/j.jhealeco.2008.10.007.

Wang, H., 2006. *Daguo weisheng zhi lun (on the health of the country)*. Beijing: Peking University Press.

Wang, S., 2011. Learning through practice and experimentation: the financing of rural health care. *In*: S. Heilmann and E.J. Perry, eds. *Mao's invisible hand: the political foundations of adaptive governance in China*. Cambridge, MA: Harvard University Press, 102–137.

Yao, K. and Wang, A., 2013. *China lets Gini out of the bottle; wide wealth gap* [online]. *Reuters*, 18 January. Available from: http://www.reuters.com/article/2013/01/18/us-china-economy-income-gap-idUSBRE90H06L20130118 [Accessed 4 February 2015].

You, X. and Kobayashi, Y., 2008. The new cooperative medical scheme in China. *Health Policy*, 91 (1), 1–9.

Appendix 1. Interview subjects

Interviews with local officials and hospital personnel

Interview code	County code	Province	Date	Institution	Position
JSAW01	A	Jiangsu	30/11/2009	County Health Bureau	Bureau Head
JSAH02	A	Jiangsu	30/11/2009	County People's Hospital	Doctor
JSBW07	B	Jiangsu	1/12/2009	County Health Bureau	Bureau Head
JSBH08	B	Jiangsu	1/12/2009	County People's Hospital	Doctor
JSCW10	C	Jiangsu	2/12/2009	County Health Bureau	Bureau Head
JSCH11	C	Jiangsu	2/12/2009	Hospital	Administrator
HNDX14	D	Hunan	14/12/2009	NCMS Office	Administrator
HNDH15	D	Hunan	14/12/2009	People's Hospital 1	Doctor
HNDH18	D	Hunan	14/12/2009	People's Hospital 2	Doctor
HNEW19	E	Hunan	15/12/2009	County Health Bureau	Bureau Head
HNEV20	E	Hunan	15/12/2009	Village Committee	Village Leader
HNEV21	E	Hunan	15/12/2009	Village	Village Head
HNEH22	E	Hunan	15/12/2009	County People's Hospital	Doctor
HNFW23	F	Hunan	17/12/2009	County Health Bureau	Administrator
HNFH24	F	Hunan	17/12/2009	County People's Hospital	Hospital Director
HNGL29	G	Hunan	14/1/2014	Office of Letters and Visits	Administrator
HNGW30	G	Hunan	14/1/2009	County Health Bureau	Bureau Head
HNGH31	G	Hunan	14/1/2009	County People's Hospital	Doctor
JSHW34	H	Jiangsu	4/3/2009	County Health Bureau	Administrator
JSHH35	H	Jiangsu	4/3/2009	County People's Hospital	Doctor
JSHH37	H	Jiangsu	4/3/2009	Village clinic	Administrator
JSIW39	I	Jiangsu	5/3/2009	County Health Bureau	Bureau Head
JSIH40	I	Jiangsu	5/3/2009	County People's Hospital	Doctor
JSIH42	I	Jiangsu	5/3/2009	Village clinic	Administrator
JSJW44	J	Jiangsu	8/3/2009	County Health Bureau	Bureau Head
JSJW45	J	Jiangsu	8/3/2009	County Health Bureau	Administrator
JSJH46	J	Jiangsu	8/3/2009	County People's Hospital	Doctor
JSKW49a	K	Jiangsu	9/3/2009	County Health Bureau	Deputy Head of Bureau
JSKW49b	K	Jiangsu	9/3/2009	County Health Bureau	Administrator

(Continued)

(Continued).

Interview code	County code	Province	Date	Institution	Position
JSKW49c	K	Jiangsu	9/3/2009	County Health Bureau	Administrator
JSKH50	K	Jiangsu	9/3/2009	County People's Hospital	Administrator
JSLW53	L	Jiangsu	10/3/2009	NCMS Office	Administrator
GSW54	M	Gansu	24/6/2010	County Health Bureau	Bureau Head
GSH55	M	Gansu	24/6/2010	Township Hospital	Managing Director
GSH56	M	Gansu	24/6/2010	Township Hospital	Hospital Director
GSW57	N	Gansu	24/6/2010	County Health Bureau	Bureau Head
GSW58	O	Gansu	29/6/2010	NCMS Office	Administrator
GSW59	P	Gansu	30/6/2010	NCMS Office	Administrator

Interviews with local officials and hospital personnel

Appendix 2. Demographic characteristics of survey respondents

Table 2.1.   Demographic characteristics of respondents.

	Jiangsu		Hubei		Yunnan		Total	
	Count	Percentage	Count	Percentage	Count	Percentage	Count	Percentage
Villagers								
Women	118	46	134	46	129	51	381	48
CCP	22	9	32	11	17	7	71	9
Ethnic minorities	0	0	28	10	47	19	75	9
Total	258	100	292	100	251	100	801	100
Village leaders								
Women	20	19	27	28	10	11	57	20
CCP	85	80	80	82	68	78	233	80
Ethnic minorities	0	0	8	8	16	18	24	8
Total	106	100	97	100	87	100	290	100

Source: Author's original survey.
Notes: One discrepancy between national demographics and our sample merits discussion: communist party membership. Communist party members comprise about 6% of the population in China (and much less in rural areas), but 9% in our sample of villagers. This slight over-representation of relatively 'elite' villagers certainly affects the inference drawn from our survey data. However, as my main research questions are related to state legitimacy and state–society relations, the over-representation of CCP members does not preclude useful analysis of these data. CCP members tend to be more politically active, more educated, but also more critical of state policies than non-CCP members. In addition, as CCP members are leaders in their communities, I expect that their views have a greater effect on other villagers and the potential for anti-government action than non-CCP members. Therefore, by including a slightly higher proportion of CCP members than is representative, our survey data more closely reflect the positions of those villagers who play a leadership role in their communities. Also, party membership is used as a control variable in my analyses; thus, I do not anticipate that this would preclude inference from our data.

Table 2.2.   Age of respondents.

	Obs.	Mean	Std. Dev.	Min.	Max.
Jiangsu					
Villagers	257	48.03	14.19	19	93
Village leaders	105	44.69	11.75	21	81
Hubei					
Villagers	290	48.26	13.81	17	87
Village leaders	97	46.46	11.79	24	86
Yunnan					
Villagers	243	43.57	16.63	17	81
Village leaders	87	45.02	8.43	25	67

Source: Author's original survey.

Table 2.3. Education level of respondents.

	Villagers		Village Leaders	
	Count	Percentage	Count	Percentage
Jiangsu				
1. No schooling	40	16	2	2
2. Primary school	64	25	5	5
3. Junior high school	90	35	20	20
4. High school	48	19	41	41
5. College and above	12	5	32	32
6. Other*	3	1	0	0
Total	257	100	100	100
Hubei				
1. No schooling	22	9	1	1
2. Primary school	77	30	5	5
3. Junior high school	117	46	35	35
4. High school	59	23	39	39
5. College and above	12	5	16	16
6. Other*	4	2	0	0
Total	291	113	96	96
Yunnan				
1. No schooling	47	18	0	0
2. Primary school	82	32	7	7
3. Junior high school	79	31	42	42
4. High school	28	11	34	34
5. College and above	15	6	4	4
6. Other*	2	1	0	0
Total	253	98	87	87

Note: *Responses to Option 6 included three graduate or professional school responses, five descriptions that were unclear, and one 'self-educated' response.
Source: Author's original survey.

Appendix 3. Villagers' ratings of local health facilities

	Villagers' ratings of local health facilities, by province					
	Jiangsu		Hubei		Yunnan	
	Count	Percentage	Count	Percentage	Count	Percentage
Village clinic						
Very poor	13	6	23	9	27	12
Poor	49	21	49	20	60	26
Middle	145	61	138	56	112	49
Good	26	11	33	13	28	12
Very good	3	1	4	2	1	0
	236	100	247	100	228	100
Township hospital						
Very poor	1	0	9	4	7	3
Poor	22	9	43	17	31	15
Middle	110	47	142	57	115	56
Good	88	37	49	20	51	25
Very good	14	6	5	2	3	1
	235	100	248	100	207	100
County hospital						
Very poor	2	1	0	0	0	0
Poor	6	3	4	2	0	0
Middle	8	3	59	25	44	21
Good	126	54	139	59	136	66
Very good	90	39	34	14	27	13
	232	100	236	100	207	100

Note: Percentages may not sum to 100 due to rounding error.
Source: Author's survey of villagers.

The development of rural primary health care in China's health system reform

Xiaoyun Liu[a], Shichao Zhao[b], Minmin Zhang[a], Dan Hu[a] and Qingyue Meng[a]

[a]China Center for Health Development Studies, Peking University, Beijing, China; [b]Center for Health Management and Policy, Shandong University, Jinan, China

China started its national health system reform in 2009, with the focus on primary health care (PHC). This study aimed to investigate the progress of PHC in rural China during the health system reform, with a special focus on human resources for health (HRH). It used data from health statistical yearbooks as well as a questionnaire survey and qualitative interviews in three provinces. The study found that central and local governments increased their financial subsidies to township health centres. Medical education and training activities were organized to improve HRH development. Health professionals' monthly income increased as a result of the implementation of a performance-based payment system. The number and quality of health professionals at township health centres had a steady increase, but health managers reported serious HRH crises in terms of attraction and retention of qualified health professionals. The amount of medical and public health services provided by township health centres had a significant increase. The study recommended the control of uncoordinated expansion of public hospitals, strengthening of medical education, and improving health professionals' income in order to promote HRH development and quality of rural PHC services.

Primary health care (PHC) is a key component of the health system. It acts as a hub from which patients are guided through the health system (WHO 2008). Having a well-functioning PHC system contributes to equity in health and health care, better service quality, and efficient use of health resources. Although PHC has been extensively studied in a well-resourced context, misunderstandings and challenges in PHC are still prevalent in low- and middle-income countries. PHC is often considered as low-tech non-professional care for the rural poor. It is often isolated from secondary and tertiary health care (WHO 2008). China has a good historical record of PHC development, especially in rural areas. But along with social and economic development, the PHC system has been considerably weakened. Since 2003, the Chinese government has been trying to re-establish the PHC system through an overall health reform plan. This article is a review of the progress of PHC reform since then by analysing data mainly collected from three provinces in eastern, central, and western China. It found that PHC has made impressive progress in China since the beginning of the health system reform. However, shortages and low quality of health professionals are the main barriers for PHC development. This study sheds light on the key challenges of China's health system reform. The policy recommendations that emerged from this study are to promote HRH development to improve rural PHC in China.

Literature review

PHC was formally promoted in the Declaration of Alma-Ata in 1978 as the key to attaining an acceptable level of health for all people in this world. One of the motivations of the PHC movement was to address the gross inequality in health status within and between countries and to promote social and economic development. PHC was considered the heart of the Health for All movement. In 1979, a new perspective of PHC, selective PHC was raised to identify and implement a package of low-cost technical interventions to tackle the main disease problems in poor countries. The debate between the two alternative options of PHC has lasted for a long time (Carrin *et al.* 2010).

The development of health policy since 1978 demonstrates that PHC has had an enormous influence on public policies, strengthening health systems, and the development of human resources for health (HRH). While there have been significant achievements, it is clear that progress towards Health for All has been uneven. The health status of some disadvantaged populations remains poor because they do not enjoy equitable, comprehensive, or even basic health care. In 2008, the World Health Report entitled 'Primary health care, now more than ever' extended a call from the World Health Organization for a global rejuvenation of PHC as an approach to strengthening health systems (WHO 2008).

The Chinese health care system has long been PHC-oriented. The community-based rural health insurance scheme (the Cooperative Medical Scheme, CMS), barefoot doctors, and the three-tier service delivery system (county hospitals, township health centres, and village clinics) formed a solid foundation for rural PHC system in the 1950s–1970s (Zhang and Unschuld 2008). The CMS was a community health insurance scheme started in the 1950s in rural China. This voluntary scheme was based on collective economy through which premiums were collected at the village level. Participants only needed to pay a very small amount of money when seeking health services. Although the benefit package was very limited, it covered both clinical and public health services. The CMS greatly helped rural residents to have equal access to basic health services.

Barefoot doctors were community health workers in rural China. The barefoot doctor system started in 1968. They were locally recruited from rural villages and received short training (3–6 months) in medicine and public health. Working in village clinics, they provided basic medical services to the rural residents and also conducted public health work. From 1968 to 1985 when China lacked qualified health workers in rural areas, barefoot doctors played important roles in providing health services to rural residents. In 1985, China stopped using the term of barefoot doctor. Most of them were transferred to village doctors as private practitioners, making a living out of drug sales based on user fees (Zhang and Unschuld 2008).

The three-tier health service delivery system including county hospitals, township health centres, and village clinics in rural areas provided basic health care to the rural population. While county hospitals were the top providers of medical services, township health centres and village clinics provided both medical and public health services. All services were covered by the CMS. Health workers from lower level health facilities had regular training and supervision from those in higher-level facilities. There was a well-functioning referral system within the three-tier service delivery structure. When patients needed to see a doctor in a county hospital, they had to be referred by doctors in township health centres, otherwise the CMS would not cover their cost.

The CMS, barefoot doctors, and three-tier service delivery system were not separate components but were well integrated into the whole rural PHC system. Barefoot doctors provided services at village clinics, the foundation of the three-tier system. All services provided in the system were covered by the CMS. The CMS also played a very important role in the referral system. The PHC system in the 1950–1970s proved to be a successful health system policy. Though rural China was relatively poor at that time, rural residents benefited from this PHC system and had equal access to basic services. This rural PHC system has greatly improved the health status of the Chinese population. The life expectancy improved from 35.0 years before 1949 to 67.9 years in 1981. The infant mortality rate dropped from around 200‰–34.7‰ in the same period. The case of rural PHC in China also contributed to the global PHC movement as an important case in the Alma-Alta Declaration in 1978 (Zhang and Unschuld 2008).

However, along with China's economic reform that started in the early 1980s, the rural PHC has been weakened. First, CMS largely collapsed as it lost its foundation of collective economy in the rural community. By the end of the 1980s, less than 10% of the Chinese rural population were covered by any health insurance scheme so that they had to pay out of pocket for their health service expenditures (Meng and Xu 2014). Second, the barefoot doctors disappeared in the same context. Most of them were transferred to village doctors as private practitioners, making a living out of drug sales based on user fees (Zhang and Unschuld 2008). Third, the referral system between the three-tier service delivery system disappeared as a result of collapse of CMS, which used to have strict requirement of mutual referral within the three tiers. At the same time, public hospitals that play a dominant role in providing secondary and tertiary health care in China went through market-oriented reforms. Public hospitals were largely self-financed through user fees. Revenues from drugs sales became the main source of public hospitals' income. Supplier-induced demand in public hospitals became a major concern. The combination of weakening PHC and expanding public hospitals had two severe conse-quences: rural population had limited access to health services and medical expenditures were significantly escalating and unaffordable (State Council 2005). The national health services survey in 2003 showed that 48.9% of patients did not seek medical care when in need. Among them, 38.2% were because of financial difficulties. About 29.6% of the patients declined doctors' advice for hospital service with the economic barrier as the top reason (70.0%). Service utilization rates were far less among non-insured patients than those with health insurance (Centre for Health Statistics and Information, Ministry of Health 2004).

In responding to this weakening rural PHC, the Chinese government initiated a series of significant reforms from the early 2000s. First, the central government decided to re-establish a New Cooperative Medical Scheme (NCMS) in 2002 (Chinese Communist Party Central Committee and State Council 2002). NCMS is a voluntary scheme, co-funded by individual premiums and government subsidies. About 20% of NCMS funds are from rural households and 80% from government subsidies. The NCMS cover-age rate increased from 10% in 2003 to 98% in 2012. The scheme is now the cornerstone of China's rural health system (Meng and Xu 2014). Second, in 2009, China started an ambitious overall health system reform (Chen 2009, Chinese Communist Party Central Committee and State Council 2009, State Council 2009). The reform includes five interdependent areas: expanding health insurance to cover more than 90% of the popula-tion, establishing a national essential medicines system to meet everyone's primary needs of medicine, improving the primary care delivery system to provide basic health care, making public health services available and equal for all, and piloting public hospital reforms (Yip *et al.* 2012).

Significance of this study

Although these five components (PHC is only one of them) are separately organized and implemented, all of them are closely related to PHC, especially in rural areas. First, basic public health services are mainly delivered by township health centres and village clinics, which may result in increased workload in public health services, and in consequence influence their functions and roles in clinical services. Second, expanding health insurance coverage affects township health centres' revenue structure (more revenue from NCMS). More importantly, with increasing financial protection and therefore higher capacity to pay for health services, service utilization of the rural population will inevitably increase. But since there is no referral and gate-keeping system in rural PHC, this increase in service utilization may occur more in hospitals than in PHC. Third, the essential medicine policy is now mainly implemented at the PHC level. This policy has a two-fold implication for township health centres and village clinics: all prescriptions have to be from the limited essential drug list and revenues from drug sales are sharply reduced as a result of the zero-markup policy. Fourth, public hospital reform may have influence on patients' choice and health workers' mobility between hospitals and PHC. Fifth, improving the PHC system includes allocating more financial resources for purchasing equipment, providing in-service training for PHC health workers, waiving tuition fees for medical students who are willing to work at township health centres after graduation, and recruiting to meet the target of one licenced physician for each township health centre by the end of 2011.

All of these reforms will have direct or indirect impact on the PHC development in rural China. This study aims to investigate the progress of PHC in rural China during the health system reform, with special focus on HRH development. It will also identify problems and challenges in PHC development in rural China and provide policy recommendations for future reform in the PHC and the overall health system.

Methods

Study design

PHC in China covers a wide range of health facilities, including community health centres and community health stations in urban areas, and township health centres and village clinics in rural areas. This article will mainly cover township health centres in rural areas.

This study takes HRH as an intermediate level between health system reform measures and PHC development in rural areas. It is based on the belief that all resource inputs in the health system and all health reform interventions can only be transferred to effective health services through the work of health professionals, with other conditions and requirement being met (Anand and Bärnighausen 2012). Therefore, this study has three components in its study design (Figure 1). It starts with describing the key reform measures related to rural PHC, with a special focus on HRH functions including education and training, and performance management. All other health system reform components including essential medicine policy, health financing reform, basic public health reform, and public hospitals reform are taken as context factors. These PHC reform measures will have an association with HRH output including number and distribution, qualification of PHC workforce, and their motivation to perform. Finally, the right number of health workers with the right skills in the right places will provide accessible and quality health services (WHO 2006). Table 1 gives the measurement indicators and their relevant data sources for each of the dimensions in the framework.

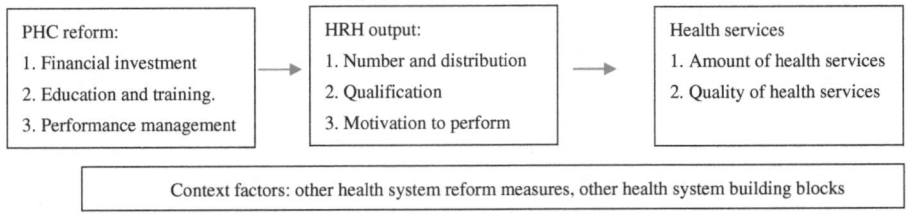

Figure 1. Conceptual framework of the study.

Source: The authors.

Table 1. Measurement and data sources.

Dimensions of PHC development	Indicators	Data sources
Financial investment	Amount of revenue sources	Facility survey
	Changes of revenue sources	Qualitative study
Education and training	Number of training activities	Questionnaire survey
	Length of training	Questionnaire survey
	Quality of training	Qualitative study
	Challenges in organizing training	Qualitative study
Performance management	Policy changes	Qualitative study
	Income level and changes	Questionnaire survey
Number of health workforce	Amount and composition of health workers	National statistics
Qualification of health workforce	Education levels	Facility survey
Motivation to perform	Motivation to perform better	Qualitative study
Amount of health services	Amount of medical and public health services	Facility survey
Quality of health services	Quality issues in health services	Qualitative study

Data sources and sampling

To answer the research questions, the study used data from three different sources. First, relevant health statistics were drawn from Chinese Health Statistics Yearbooks, including number and qualification of the health workforce, and amount of health service at PHC levels (National Committee of Health and Family Planning 2013). Second, a survey was conducted in three provinces. Health professional from township health centres were invited to complete questionnaires. Third, qualitative interviews were also conducted in the three provinces. In the following are the sampling process and data collection methods in the three provinces.

The three provinces were selected using a purposive sampling method. Shandong Province represents the more developed area in eastern China, Anhui Province, located in central China, represents the middle level development, and Shaanxi Province represents the less developed areas in western China. In each province, three counties were selected, representing different socioeconomic development levels within the province. In each county, five township health centres were selected for this study. The selection of township health centres was based on two criteria: (1) staff size of the township health centres, two were bigger (referred to as central township health centres), three were smaller (ordinary township health centres) and (2) the township health centres should be evenly located in terms of distance in the county.

Data collection

A field survey was conducted in August 2013. In each township health centre, health professionals who were available at the day of investigation were invited to complete a questionnaire. Four types of health professionals were included in the survey: doctors, nurses, technicians, and public health workers. The contents of the survey were comprehensive, but for this article, related contents included health professionals' geographic information, their income level, and the training they received during the last year. The respondents were invited to a meeting room within the township health centre to complete the survey. The questionnaires were self-administered, but there were graduate students in public health from Peking University available to explain the requirement of the survey and answer any questions they raised during the survey. Each completed questionnaire was carefully checked by the graduate students on the spot. Any identified mistakes and missing answers were corrected before the respondent left. In total, 803 complete questionnaires were collected in the three provinces (Table 1). Each township health centre also filled out a facility questionnaire including information about the centre's income structure.

Qualitative interviews with health managers and frontline health workers were conducted. The interviewees included managers from county health bureaus and township health centres and health workers from township health centres (doctors, nurses, technicians, and public health workers). Contents in the topic guides included implementation of PHC reform activities, especially on education and training, performance management, HRH attraction, and retention. The interviews were usually conducted in the offices of the interviewees. Other irrelevant persons except for the interviewee were asked to leave the room to make sure the interview was not interrupted. With informed consent, all interviews were tape-recorded. Interviewers were researchers from Peking University, while the note-takers were usually graduate students in public health. In total, 190 interviews were conducted (Table 2).

Data processing and analysis

Questionnaire survey data were double input with consistency check. SPSS (20.0) was applied to analyse the data. We mainly used descriptive methods to compare the means and proportions of various indicators between different years and different cadres.

Table 2. Sample description of surveys and interviews.

	Shandong	Anhui	Shaanxi	Total
Health professional survey				
Doctors	78	110	50	238
Nurses	50	74	43	167
Public health workers	87	66	33	186
Technicians	55	114	43	212
Sub-total	270	364	169	803
Individual interviews				
County health bureau managers	3	3	2	8
THC managers	14	15	15	44
Doctors	17	15	17	49
Nurses	15	15	14	44
Public health workers	15	15	15	45
Sub-total	64	63	63	190

Transcriptions of qualitative interviews were analysed using MaxQDA (11.0). A thematic framework was developed based on the interview topic guides and emerging issues from the interview. The thematic framework is consistent with Figure 1, including topics on financial subsidies to township health centres, education and training of health professionals, performance appraisal and remuneration, and attraction and retention, among others. Using MaxQDA, two researchers independently coded the transcripts based on the thematic framework. The coded segments were then retrieved, grouped into a table and summarized accordingly (Spencer *et al.* 2003).

Results

Financial subsidies

Before the health system reform, township health centres heavily relied on user fees to cover their operational cost, especially revenues from drug sales. Since 2009, the financial arrangement of township health centres has had significant changes. The most important change was related to the essential medicine policy. Due to the zero markup policy, township health centres can no longer make any profit from drug sales and therefore lost their major revenue source. Local governments provided special subsidies to compensate township health centres for their loss due to the essential medicine policy. But township health centre managers reported during the interviews that this compensation can hardly cover their financial loss.

The second change in financial arrangement is about basic public health services. The central and local government input 25 yuan per resident to purchase basic public health services. This fund was directly allocated to township health centres who should further allocate 40% of the fund to village clinics. Many township health centre directors reported that this fund became a major source of their income. Other government subsidies to township health centres included personnel salary, special fund for building construction, and for purchasing equipment.

Although township health centre directors repeatedly complained about their financial loss due to the essential medicine policy, the quantitative financial information collected from the selected 45 township centres in the three provinces was not as bad as what they reported in the qualitative interviews. Table 3 shows that the total income of a township

Table 3. Average income per township health centre in three provinces (10,000 yuan).

	2008	2010	2012
Total income	319.4	398.8	593.5
Shandong	324.4	443.8	684.3
Anhui	286.9	414.8	664.7
Shanxi	253.2	393.2	525.2
1. Government subsidy	59.3	155.3	260.7
1.1 Personnel salary	37.6	86.8	137.6
1.2 Subsidy for basic public health services	6.7	51.3	95.5
1.3 Building construction and purchasing of equipment	10.3	6.9	4.9
2. Income from medical services	97.7	89.4	142.5
3. Income from drug sales	129.3	120.7	178.3
4. Other income	33.1	33.4	12

Source: Health facility survey.

health centres had an 85.5% increase in 2012 over 2008. The increase of overall govern-ment subsidies between 2008 and 2012 was 4.4 times, mainly on personnel salary and basic public health services. Medical services income had a steady increase (45.9%) over the 4 years' period. Income from drug sales had a slight decrease in 2010 when the essential medicine policy was initially implemented and increased again in 2012.

Training

Health professionals reported that more training activities were organized during the health system reform in order to strengthen health professionals' skills and ability (Table 4). A doctor in 2010 could have 2.54 times of training activities on average. This number increased to 4.69 in 2012. Compared to 2010, nurses and public health workers had nearly twice the training opportunities in 2012 than in 2010. However, further analysis showed that the majority of the trainings were only very short ones. In 2012, among the 4.69 times of training activities for doctors, 2.74 times (58.4%) were only 1-day training.

During the qualitative interviews, respondents reported three issues regarding the in-service trainings. First, the effects of some short trainings were not satisfactory. The main training approach was lecturing, with very limited practice. Second, with increasing training activities, township health centres had difficulties in selecting and sending people to attend the training. The main reason was that sending people to attend training would affect their daily service provision. In some special cases, township health centres would select the same health worker to attend various training activities. Third, another challenge township health centres faced was the concern about staff loss after training. Some township health centre directors reported such cases. When they sent doctors to county hospitals to receive training, some may find job opportunities in the county hospitals after training.

Targeted education programme

Since 2010, along with the overall health system reform, China has implemented a national programme to train health professionals for rural health facilities. The programme

Table 4. Number of training activities for health workers in township health centres in three provinces.

	Doctors	Nurses	Public health workers
2010	2.54	3.81	4.99
2012	4.69	7.56	7.28
Length of training in 2012			
1 day	2.74	4.16	4.94
2–3 days	0.76	0.5	1.13
4 days–4 week	0.24	0.9	0.35
1–2 weeks	0.19	0.53	0.24
3–4 weeks	0.14	0.67	0.19
1–3 months	0.19	0.28	0.14
3 months–1 year	0.31	0.46	0.24
More than 1 year	0.12	0.06	0.05

Source: Health professional questionnaire survey.
Note: Information about training opportunities was not available for technicians.

has been mainly implemented in the less developed central and western provinces of China. Based on local demand from county health authorities, medical universities have targeted recruitment of medical students with rural backgrounds. After signing a contract with local health authorities, these recruited students have a waiver of tuition fee with additional living allowances. They will receive 5-year medical training in medical universities or colleges, with a focus on general practice. In return for this financial support, medical graduates from this programme will have to observe the contract and work in their rural hometown for 6 years. The programme is funded by the central government. Concerns were raised among policymakers and health managers about the effects of this programme, as the first group of medical students admitted in 2010 will soon graduate in 2015 after 5 years' medical education. One of the major concerns is that how many of these students will observe the contract to work and practice in their rural hometown, and whether they will stay there for 6 years as the programme requires.

Performance-based payment

In 2009, township health centres began to implement performance-based salary. Local governments took the main financial responsibility to cover the health staff's salary at township health centres. The total salary is divided into two parts: basic salary and performance salary. The performance salary usually makes up about 30–40% of the total salary, which is floating based on performance appraisal. As a result of this salary reform, the salary level at township health centres increased. Table 5 shows that all four types of health cadres had an annual increase of 160–219 yuan per month between 2012 and 2013, with nurses having the biggest increase.

Although the questionnaire survey found a modest increase of monthly income, satisfaction about the current income level among health professionals was very low. About 67.1% health professionals reported they were not satisfied with the current income.

One major issue reported during the qualitative interviews about the performance based payment was about incentive and motivation. Health professionals reflected that although part of the salary should be linked to performance, in practice, everybody nearly got the same income regardless of their efforts and workload. One explanation of this by township health centre managers was to avoid unfairness. As a result, after implementing the performance-based salary system, many health workers were less motivated to provide medical services. Township health managers were aware of this concern, but were also worried about the potential conflicts if income differences between different staff members were too big. They were exploring optimal performance appraisal mechanisms.

Table 5. Monthly income of health professionals at township health centres (yuan) in three provinces.

	2013	2012	Increase
Doctors	2457 ± 706	2294 ± 759	163
Nurses	2166 ± 874	1947 ± 762	219
Public health workers	2202 ± 710	2032 ± 669	170
Technicians	2184 ± 715	2004 ± 672	180

Source: Health professional questionnaire survey.

Changes in HRH in rural PHC

We collected data from national health statistics yearbooks to reflect the changing trend of HRH at township health centres since the beginning of the health system reform. Table 6 shows that all types of health professionals at township health centres had a steady increase between 2008 and 2012. The total number of health professionals had an 18.2% increase over the 4 years.

The qualification of health professionals at township health centres was rather low. Only 6.1% of health professionals had a university degree. The majority of them only had 2–3 years medical education from technical secondary schools. However, health professionals' qualifications have been increasing over the last years. In 2005, only 2.2% had a university degree. In terms of their technical title, the majority of them only had a primary technical title. Only 0.9% had a senior-level technical title. There were no significant changes between 2005 and 2012 in their technical titles (Table 7).

Qualitative interviews in the three provinces portrayed a different picture in terms of HRH development at township health centres. Almost all health managers reported that township health centre faced HRH crises. They had great difficulties in attracting new staff, especially those with a university degree. Loss of health professionals was reported to be very serious. The main barriers for attraction and retention of HRH

Table 6. Number of health professionals per township health centre (2008–2012).

	2008	2010	2012
Health professional	23.52	26.03	27.82
Licenced physician	6.30	6.70	6.67
Licenced assistant physician	4.24	4.6	4.9
Registered nurse	4.88	5.82	6.77
Pharmacist	1.89	1.96	1.98
Technician	1.24	1.38	1.43
Other	4.96	5.57	6.07
Number of health professionals at THC per 1000 rural population	1.22	1.30	1.37

Source: National Committee of Health and Family Planning (2013).

Table 7. Professional qualification of health workers in township health centre (%).

	2005	2010	2011	2012
Education level				
University and above	2.2	5.7	5.9	6.1
Junior college	20.3	33.9	34.8	35.7
Technical secondary school	58.7	52.2	51.8	51.3
Secondary school or below	18.7	8.3	7.5	6.8
Technical title				
Senior level	0.8	0.9	0.9	0.9
Middle level	13.0	14.0	13.5	13.1
Primary level	86.2	85.1	85.6	86.0

Source: National Committee of Health and Family Planning (2013).

included low income, limited career development opportunities, family issues, and others. A township health centre director in Shaanxi Province said: 'in the last 6–7 years, we lost a dozen good health workers. Most of them are young people. They require a better working environment. Many of them went to county hospitals. I feel a township health center is only a transit place for them.' A county health bureau director in Shandong Province reported: 'Township health centers had more and more difficulties to attract high level talents. The first reason is low income. But the remote location is a more important reason; township health center are usually 30–40 kilometers from the county.'

Changes in service delivery in PHC

Table 8 shows the changing trends of medical services (outpatient visits and inpatient admissions) and public health services at township health centres in the three provinces between 2008 and 2012. Compared to 2008, the amount of outpatient services per township health centre in 2012 significantly increased in all three provinces, while the changing trends of inpatient services showed variations among the three provinces. In Shandong Province, the number of inpatient admissions decreased between 2008 and 2012. Anhui Province witnessed a decrease of inpatient services in 2010, but then an increase in 2012. Township health centres in Shaanxi Province had a smaller number of inpatient admissions compared to other two provinces, but had a steady increase.

In terms of public health work, township health centres reported a sharp increase of workload covering many different public health activities. Table 8 also shows the increasing trend of some selected indicators in public health services.

Qualitative interviews reflected some important changes in service delivery at township health centres. First, township health centres' workload in providing basic public health services had a significant increase. Some clinical doctors and nurses reported that they also needed to do public health work. Second, health managers said that township health centres were losing some of their abilities in clinical service provision, for example, minor surgeries and attending birth delivery. Third, there was very limited information available about the quality of both clinical and public health services they provided at township health centres.

Discussion

This study drew on different data sources to investigate the progress of PHC in rural China since 2009. There are a few limitations of this study. The main data source is from the field survey of three provinces: Shandong, Anhui, and Shaanxi. These three provinces were selected to represent eastern, central, and western China, yet they may not be able to represent the whole country. Furthermore, for some indicators, we also drew on national data. There may be some discrepancy between the national situation and the cases in the three provinces. Any generalization of the findings to the whole country should be conducted with caution.

Second, the study found that health system reforms have deployed many specific interventions on PHC in rural China, including government financial subsidies, education and training for HRH, and performance management. HRH at township health centres has been increasing since the health system reform in 2009, though directors of township heath centres and county health bureaus believe that township health centres are still facing severe HRH challenges. The amount of both outpatient and inpatient services

Table 8. Volume of medical and public health services per township health centre in three provinces.

	Shandong			Anhui			Shaanxi		
	2008	2010	2012	2008	2010	2012	2008	2010	2012
Outpatient visits	30087	37959	55195	44732	34991	39107	6128	12726	10081
Inpatient admissions	2556	1438	1154	1081	817	1156	220	230	361
Number of medical records made	5250	29360	41140	343	12219	31356	7063	12787	16774
Number of health education documents circulated	5836	30750	40443	2000	18003	22810	5060	7664	38649
Number of antenatal visits	215	333	426	192	469	537	199	238	274
Number of postnatal visits	237	341	423	171	369	500	198	236	275
% of hypertension patients under management	0	71	79	0.3	87.6	86	56	88	98
% of diabetes patients under management	25	73	76.1	0	82.2	84	64.3	85.7	97.2

Source: Health facility survey.

provided at the township level went up in the last few years; however, higher-level public hospitals saw a much faster increase in patient volume.

The quantitative and qualitative results about HRH development at township health centres showed contradictory pictures. While the quantitative data indicated that both the amount and qualification of health professionals at the township level have been improving, respondents complained that township health centres have been losing their talented health professionals and have great difficulties in attracting new ones. There are two potential reasons behind this paradox. First, with the economic development and expanding coverage of NCMS, rural residents' demands for health services are largely released. This can be reflected by the fact that both outpatient and inpatient services rapidly increased in the last few years. This increasing demand for health services implies increasing demand for HRH. Additionally, more financial input into township health centres and new technologies and equipment also exacerbate township health centres' thirst for more qualified health professionals. The modest increase in HRH may not be sufficient to meet their rapidly increasing requirement. Second, with the expansion of public hospitals, more doctors and nurses are needed at these higher-level hospitals. This will inevitably promote the mobility of high-quality health workers from township health centres to public hospitals. Although township health centres may recruit some young health workers to compensate for the loss, the imbalance between staff loss and new recruitments still creates huge challenges for township health centres to develop their HRH.

Although PHC in rural China has been developing during the health system reform, the disparity between PHC and public hospitals is enlarging. Rural residents' capacity to pay for health services have increased due to the NCMS development, and many of them bypass the township health centres to seek better quality health care at county hospitals or even high level hospitals. If this new phenomenon is not taken into consideration, PHC in rural China may be weakened in the long run. Fortunately, the central government is promptly responding to this and recently issued an urgent notice to control the uncoordinated expansion of public hospitals (NCHFP 2014).

Controlling public hospitals' expansion does not automatically bring better development of PHC. This study concludes that the key driving force to improve PHC is the quality of health services and HRH development. The study presents two recommendations to improve HRH development in rural PHC. First, the government should strengthen medical education to cultivate more qualified health professionals for PHC. The targeted education programme with compulsory rural service is one of the options. As they are graduating soon, comprehensive administrative measures should be put in place to make sure they observe the contract to serve the rural health enterprise after graduation. Second, rural jobs lack attraction to medical graduates and health professionals due to the low income level and many other barriers. Considerable rural allowances should be added to the current salary system to improve the attraction and retention of the rural health workforce.

Acknowledgement
Thanks to Dr Edward C. Mignot, Shandong University, for linguistic advice.

Disclosure statement
No potential conflict of interest was reported by the authors.

References

Anand, S. and Bärnighausen, T., 2012. Health workers at the core of the health system: framework and research issues. *Health Policy*, 105, 185–191. doi:10.1016/j.healthpol.2011.10.012

Carrin, G., *et al.*, 2010. *Health systems policy, finance, and organization*. New York, NY: Academic Press.

Centre for Health Statistics and Information, Ministry of Health, 2004. *An analysis report on National Health Services Survey 2003*. Beijing: Centre for Health Statistics and Information, Ministry of Health.

Chen, Z., 2009. Launch of the health-care reform plan in China. *The Lancet*, 373, 1322–1324. doi:10.1016/S0140-6736(09)60753-4

Chinese Communist Party Central Committee and State Council, 2002. *Decisions on the strengthening of the rural health system [Official Document No. 13]*. Beijing: Chinese Communist Party Central Committee and State Council.

Chinese Communist Party Central Committee and State Council, 2009. *The standing conference of State Council of China adopted guidelines for furthering the reform of health-care system in principle*. Beijing: Chinese Communist Party Central Committee and State Council.

Meng, Q. and Xu, K., 2014. Progress and challenges of the rural cooperative medical scheme in China. *Bulletin of the World Health Organization*, 92, 447–451. doi:10.2471/BLT.13.131532

National Committee of Health and Family Planning, 2013. *Health statistics year book 2013*. Beijing: National Committee of Health and Family Planning.

National Committee of Health and Family Planning, 2014. *Urgent notice to control the rapid expansion of public hospitals*. Beijing: National Committee of Health and Family Planning.

Spencer, L., Ritchie, J., and O'Connor, W., 2003. Carrying out qualitative analysis. *In*: J. Ritchie and J. Lewis, eds. *Qualitative research practice: a guide for social science students and researchers*. London: Sage, 219–262.

State Council, 2005. *China health system reform*. Beijing: State Council.

State Council, 2009. *Current major project on health care system reform (2009–2011)*. Beijing: State Council.

World Health Organization, 2006. *World health organization report 2006-working together for health*. Geneva: World Health Organization.

World Health Organization, 2008. *World health organization report 2008-primary health care (now more than ever)*. Geneva: World Health Organization.

Yip, W.C.-M., *et al.*, 2012. Early appraisal of China's huge and complex health-care reforms. *The Lancet*, 379, 833–842. doi:10.1016/S0140-6736(11)61880-1

Zhang, D. and Unschuld, P.U., 2008. China's barefoot doctor: past, present, and future. *The Lancet*, 372 (9653), 1865–1867. doi:10.1016/S0140-6736(08)61355-0

The impact of China's Zero-Markup Drug Policy on county hospital revenue and government subsidy levels

Zhongliang Zhou[a], Yanfang Su[b], Benjamin Campbell[c], Zhiying Zhou[d], Jianmin Gao[a], Qiang Yu[e], Jiuhao Chen[f] and Yishan Pan[g]

[a]School of Public Policy and Administration, Xi'an Jiaotong University, Xi'an, China; [b]Department of Global Health and Population, Harvard School of Public Health, Boston, MA, USA; [c]Department of Anthropology, Dartmouth College, Hanover, NH, USA; [d]School of Public Health, Xi'an Jiaotong University Health Science Center, Xi'an, China; [e]Ankang Municipal Development and Reform Commission, Ankang, China; [f]Ningshan County Hospital, Shaanxi, China; [g]Zhenping County Hospital, Shaanxi, China

In 2009, the Chinese government passed the Zero-Markup Drug Policy, which strives to contain the costs of medicines and ultimately reduce the financial burden to the public, especially those in low-income settings. This study aims to evaluate the impact of the Zero-Markup Drug Policy on health care provision, revenue structures in county hospitals, and demand for fiscal compensation from the government. Our study employs a difference-in-difference model to measure the difference in several indicators between two hospitals, Ningshan County Hospital, which implemented the policy, and Zhenping County Hospital, which had not. The main indicators include health care provision, drug revenue as a part of total hospital revenue, and level of government subsidy. The data come from hospital financial statements and operation reports. The findings of the study show that for Ningshan County Hospital the zero-markup policy led to an increase in health care provision and a sustained total hospital income despite a decrease in drug revenue. The enhancement in outpatient and inpatient visits also represents progress from the lens of the government, whose mission is to ensure greater access to care for the population. The study demonstrates that with minimal or no subsidy, the government can catalyse the zero-markup policy and potentially generate positive outcomes for county hospitals.

1. Introduction

China has initiated ambitious health reforms since 2009. At the heart of this movement has been the reconstruction of a national primary health care system as well as a bolstering of insurance programmes targeting low-income citizens (Süssmuth-Dyckerhoff and Wang 2010). Specifically, the New Cooperative Medical Schemes (NCMS) substantially increased the level of health insurance coverage for the poor. Furthermore, the Chinese central government declared that the development of a national essential medicines system was a top priority in the reforms (The State Council of China 2009). This effort was strengthened by the National Essential Medicines Policy, which strives to make cost-effective medicines more accessible (WHO 2001).

Zhongliang Zhou and Yanfang Su joint first authorship.

Despite these efforts to broaden health coverage and availability of essential drugs, health goods and services remain largely inaccessible and unaffordable to the most vulnerable populations. For example, a recent study revealed health inequity in rural China, where inpatient care utilization has been largely pro-rich between 1993 and 2008 (Zhou *et al.* 2013). One of the primary drivers of this inequity is the cost of drugs, which can pose a significant burden on low-income people. As increasing empirical evidence shows, drug costs are the primary reason for medical impoverishment in rural China (Hu *et al.* 2007). This potentially impoverishing burden of drug costs is especially precarious for patients with chronic conditions, who need to make frequent visits to the hospital and can incur absorbent medication costs that are not covered under the NCMS, the predominant health coverage scheme. A study by Yip and Hsiao found that among all rural poor households, 11.6% became impoverished as a result of outpatient expenses related to chronic disease (Yip and Hsiao 2009). In an effort to address the financial burden experienced by patients in rural settings, the country strives to match its early success in 'broadening' health coverage with a major 'deepening' of health care (Eggleston 2012).

A fundamental component of 'deepening' health care is ensuring that essential drugs are affordable for even the most vulnerable patients (Gulliford *et al.* 2002). To achieve this, the Chinese government passed the Zero-Markup Policy for Essential Drugs, which sets ambitious goals to contain the costs of medicines and ultimately reduce the financial burden to the public, especially those in low-income settings. This policy can have far-reaching effects, and this paper specifically aims to explore the ramifications of the policy on hospital revenue structures as well as the extent of government involvement through subsidies.

The revenue of public hospitals in China mainly consists of fiscal compensation (subsidies from the government), medical revenue (medical fees, examination fees, test fees, surgery fees, bed fees, etc.), and drug revenue (Yao *et al.* 2003). However, since the implementation of Reform and Opening-up policy in 1978, the proportion of the fiscal compensation out of total revenue in public hospitals has been decreasing year by year. In 2009, the proportion of fiscal compensation out of total revenue was merely 10% (Ministry of Health 2010). With the decreasing proportion of fiscal compensation primarily from 1986 to 2002 (National Bureau of Statistics of China 2004), drug sales gradually became the major source of revenue for hospitals. In China, hospitals are allowed to sell drugs at 15% markup. In 2009, drug revenue reached 43% of the total revenue in public hospitals, which is about 20% higher than the average percentage among the Organisation for Economic Co-operation and Development (OECD) countries (OECD 2013). This phenomenon of 'yi yao yang yi' – compensation for hospital medical costs through drug-selling profits – results in the rapid increase of medical costs for patients. From 1993 to 2008, the per-visit outpatient and inpatient expenses in public medical institutions had increased by 1126% and 442%, respectively (Center for Health Statistics and Information and MOH 1994, 2009). By the end of 2009, the per-visit outpatient and inpatient expenses were 155 Yuan and 5897 Yuan, respectively, in which the drug expenses accounted for 60% and 46%, respectively (Ministry of Health 2010).

'Yi yao yang yi' poses a great threat to achieving one of China's overarching health system reform goals, namely, ensuring access to affordable care for all. In order to alleviate the phenomenon of 'yi yao yang yi' and decrease the proportion of drug costs in medical expenses, the Chinese government issued 'the Suggestions of CPC Central Committee and the State Council on Deepening the Reform of the Health care System' in April, 2009, which clearly stated that the policy of drug sale with additional markup should be gradually eliminated in public hospitals. In its place should be a policy of zero-markup in drug sales.

Since 2009, the zero-markup drug policy has been implemented primarily in primary health care institutions in China. A review of the literature shows that the policy of zero-markup in drug sales reduces the reliance of primary care institutions on drug revenue to compensate for the deficit in overall medical revenue (Li *et al.* 2008, He *et al.* 2011). A plethora of other recent studies has also shown that, at the level of primary health care institutions, the policy has led to several key advancements. Firstly, the policy has been shown to increase the provision of outpatient services. Using data from 20 community health institutions, Tao's study (2011) shows that the outpatient provision increased by 25% after the implementation of the zero-markup policy. Chen *et al.* (2010) also found that the zero-markup policy increased the outpatient provision in township hospitals and community health care centres. While increased health care provision represents progress, additional research has shown that perhaps one negative outcome of increased provision has been that it may actually result in decreased drug availability (Fang *et al.* 2013). Secondly, the zero-markup drug policy has led to changes in facility revenue streams. One study conducted by Jin *et al.* (2010) shows that as a result of zero-markup policies, revenue from drug sales deceased in Shanghai's primary medical institutions; however, the total revenue remained relatively unchanged due to increased subsidies from the government. In addition, Chen *et al.* (2010) found an increasing trend of medical revenue for the community medical institutions after implementation of the zero-markup policy. Furthermore, Lang and Li (2010) indicated that although the drug revenue decreased in the community medical institutions after the implementation of zero-markup policy, the drug revenue was still 63% of the total revenue. Thirdly, research has shown that zero-markup policy at the level of the primary care institutions did not change the number of medicines per prescription (Yang *et al.* 2012).

Although the zero-markup policy has proven to be effective in primary health care institutions, the phenomenon of 'yi yao yang yi' persists in public hospitals at the county levels and higher levels. County public hospitals are the main provider of health care in rural China and they undertake the vital task of treating patients with common medical conditions. More than 48% of patient hospitalizations occur at county hospitals, according to the fourth National Health Service Survey. From a cost perspective, statistics from the Ministry of Health in China show that expenses incurred by county hospitals comprise approximately 40% of the total medical expenses among all medical institutions in the rural areas (Ministry of Health 2011). To curb the rising costs of health care in rural China, then, it would be strategic to focus on county hospitals. The policy of zero-markup in essential drugs has been piloted at some county hospitals in some provinces. In September 2011, Fuyang County and 28 other counties in Zhejiang were selected as the pilot sites to implement a zero-markup policy. Furthermore, in June 2011, Shaanxi province announced the initiation of a 'Plan of Centralized Purchase of Medicine in Public Hospitals', and piloted the zero-markup policy in county hospitals. The shift to implement the zero-markup policy in county hospitals is imperative and reflects efforts at 'deepening' health system reform in China.

However, scientific programme evaluation has not been conducted to assess the impact of this policy on health care provision, revenue structures in public hospitals, and the demand for fiscal compensation from the government. This study aims to evaluate the zero-markup policy from the perspective of county hospitals and the government. As mentioned, most research on the effect of the policy of zero-markup on drug sales in China has focused on the community-level medical institutions. This study, in contrast, assesses the zero-markup policy at the county hospital level in the following areas: (1) analysing the effects of the zero-markup policy on health service provision; and (2) analysing the effects of the zero-markup policy on hospital revenue and fiscal compensation.

This study aims to fill important research gaps. First, because nearly all prior research focuses on the community-level medical institutions, this study aims to contribute to the literature on evaluations of the zero-markup policy at the level of county hospitals. Second, most previous research only collected data in the treatment group to conduct pre–post comparison, which lacks scientific rigor in evaluating the policy. In order to overcome the limitations in the previous research, the current study evaluates two public county-level hospitals, in which one hospital has implemented the zero-markup policy (treatment group) and the other has not implemented the policy (control group). In Section 2, the study methodology will be discussed. Section 3 will uncover the results, with specific attention to the impact of the zero-markup policy on health care provision and hospital medical revenue as well as fiscal compensation. The results are discussed and interpreted in Section 4. In this section, the limitations of the study are also presented. Lastly, Section 5 concludes with summary points and policy recommendations.

2. Methods

2.1. Study design

With the hospital as the unit of analysis, a difference-in-difference (DID) model was used to evaluate the effects of the zero-markup policy on several key indicators, including health care provision and hospital revenue. Variation in these variables was measured between the treatment-group hospital and control-group hospital in a pre–post manner. In addition, we used two methods to estimate the specific amount of government subsidy required to incentivize hospital implementation of the zero-markup policy.

In policy research, the availability of study samples is essential. Although this study measures change over only two years for two county hospitals, the DID method was selected as a more informative strategy than the case study method. Despite the limited sample size, the internal validity of the study design is enhanced by documenting the historical trend from 2007 to 2010 for both the treatment-group and control-group hospitals. This allows for an informative, although limited, causal inference about the effect of the policy.

2.2. Study fields

The site selected for this study was Ningshan County Hospital in Ankang city, Shaanxi province. The zero-markup policy was implemented in Ningshan County Hospital on 1 December 2010. At this hospital, 44% of essential drugs were selected to be subject to the zero-markup policy. From 1 December 2010 to 11 November 2011, the total cost of drugs purchased by Ningshan County Hospital was 7.88 million and the total revenue of the drugs sold by the hospital was 6.96 million. From this total, the cost and revenue of zero-markup drugs were 1.27 million and 1.1 million, respectively, accounting for 16.12% and 15.8% of the total cost and revenue. Although the proportion of essential drugs was 44%, the revenue from essential drugs was less than 44%, indicating that the unit prices of essential drugs are lower than that of the other drugs.

Zhenping County Hospital in Shaanxi province was selected as the control group for several important reasons. First, both Ningshan County and Zhenping County are administrated by the Ankang municipal government. As the pilot county, Ningshan County started to implement the policy of zero-markup in drug sale since the end of 2010, but Zhenping County did not implement the zero-markup policy until 2012. Other social policies made by provincial government and municipal government were similar in the two counties. Second, both Ningshan County and Zhenping County are located in similar mountainous regions. Ningshan County is located in the south foot of Qin Mountain and Zhenping County is located in the north foot of Daba Mountain. The existence of parallel terrains in the two counties suggests that rural residents face similar challenges in terms of access to health care. Third, the health resources in Ningshan County and Zhenping County are similar. There are 14 township health care centres, 98 village clinics, 275 beds for hospitalization, and 308 health care professionals in Ningshan County, compared with 12 township level health centres, 78 village clinics, 242 beds for hospitalization, and 199 health care professionals in Zhenping County. The numbers of hospitalization beds are similar in the two hospitals, which are 151 and 150, respectively. Fourth, the clinical departments of the two hospitals are similar.

2.3. Data

Data used in this study include the hospitals' basic facility information, the financial statements, and the operation reports. The hospitals' basic facility information includes the hospital certificate, department names, number of staff, and number of beds in both Ningshan and Zhenping County hospitals. The financial statements include the two hospitals' revenue, the composition of revenue, and expenditure from 2007 to 2011. The operation reports include the two hospitals' outpatient and inpatient provision records from 2007 to 2011.

2.4. Analytical methods

2.4.1. Difference in difference

The DID method was used to analyse the effects of the zero-markup policy (Wooldridge 2005). As seen in Equation (1), $y_{1,0}$ is the evaluation indicator for treatment-group hospital in 2010, $y_{0,0}$ is the evaluation indicator for the control-group hospital in 2010, $y_{1,1}$ is the evaluation indicator for the treatment-group hospital in 2011, and $y_{0,1}$ is the evaluation indicator for the control-group hospital in 2011. Therefore, the implementation effect of zero-markup policy is

$$\beta = (y_{1,1} - y_{1,0}) - (y_{0,1} - y_{0,0}) \tag{1}$$

In Equation (1), the first subscript '1' means treatment-group hospital and '0' means control-group hospital; the second subscript '1' means the year of 2011 and '0' means the year of 2010. Coefficient β indicates the effect of the zero-markup policy. DID is based on the assumption that the trends of target indicators between treatment-group and control-group hospitals are similar to each other without the policy intervention. This study will test whether the assumption is satisfied in the beginning of the results.

2.4.2. Estimating the government subsidy

In order to answer the question of how much fiscal revenue should be allocated to implement the zero-markup policy, two estimation methods were employed in this study. First, as the current practice, the Chinese government estimates the appropriate hospital subsidy after accounting for the previous markup in drug retail prices by 15%. The information with regard to total drug revenue and the proportion of the revenue of zero-markup drug out of total drug revenue in 2011 was collected from Ningshan County Hospital. Equation (2) shows how government subsidy is computed using this method:

$$\begin{aligned} \text{Government subsidy} = {}&\text{total drug revenue} \\ &\times \text{proportion of revenue of zero-markup drug out of total drug revenue} \qquad (2) \\ &\times \text{the markup rate in drug sale} \end{aligned}$$

Second, it is critiqued in this study that the above method using the 15% markup principle neglects the fact that the zero-markup policy does increase hospital health care revenue. Alternatively, government subsidy could be estimated by the 'natural growth principle'. Specifically, Equation (3) was used to more accurately measure government subsidy:

$$\begin{aligned} \text{Percentage increase of health care revenue} = {}&(\text{health care revenue in 2011} \\ &- \text{health care revenue in 2010})/\text{health care revenue in 2010} \end{aligned} \qquad (3)$$

Setting natural growth of health care revenue at 5% annually, government compensates the hospitals if hospital health care revenue increases less than 5% after implementing the zero-markup drug policy; when the hospitals reach natural growth rate or exceed the rate, government does not subsidize the hospitals. This is the rationale for using the 'natural growth principle' to determine whether the government should subsidize the hospitals.

3. Results

3.1. Testing the assumption of DID

The DID method is based on the assumption that, without the implementation of the intervention of interest, the trend of the outcome variables from treatment group and control group should be similar. Figures 1–4 show that, for per-visit outpatient expense, per-visit inpatient expense, and inpatient service provision, the trend in Ningshan County Hospital is similar to that in Zhenping County Hospital from 2007 to 2010, thus substantiating the hypothesis of DID. Figures 1–4 also show that the trend for the treated county, Ningshan, was interfered by the zero-markup policy in 2011. Therefore, DID is a valid method to be used in evaluating the effects of zero-markup policy on per-visit medical expense and medical service provision in these county hospitals.

From Figures 5 and 6, we find that the trends of total health care revenue and the proportion of drug revenue in total health care revenue are similar in Ningshan and Zhenping County hospitals. However, after the implementation of zero-markup policy in 2010, the proportion of drug revenue in total health care revenue in Ningshan County Hospital declined significantly, compared with the increase of the proportion in Zhenping County Hospital between 2010 and 2011.

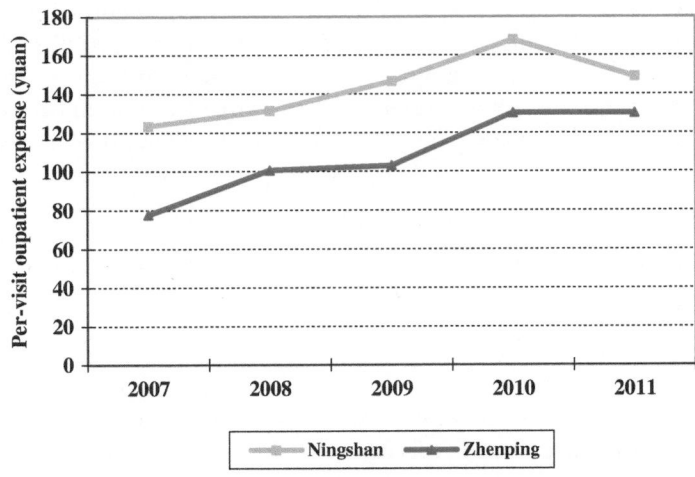

Figure 1. The trends of per-visit outpatient expense in Ningshan and Zhenping County hospitals from 2007 to 2011. Data source: Annual operation reports from 2007 to 2011 in Ningshan and Zhenping County hospitals.

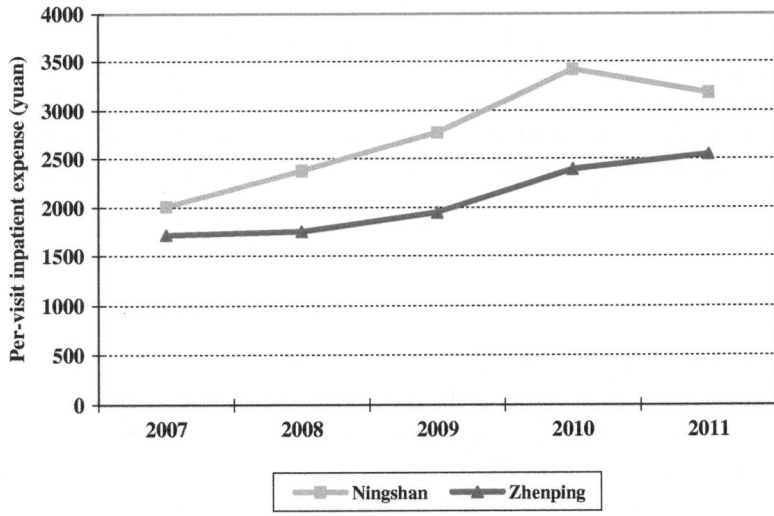

Figure 2. The trends of per-visit inpatient expense in Ningshan and Zhenping County hospitals from 2007 to 2011. Data source: Annual operation reports from 2007 to 2011 in Ningshan and Zhenping County hospitals.

3.2. The effects of zero-markup on medical expense per visit

From the results of DID in Table 1, with the implementation of zero-markup policy in Ningshan County Hospital, the per-visit outpatient expense and the per-visit inpatient expense dropped by 19.02 Yuan and 389.11 Yuan, respectively.

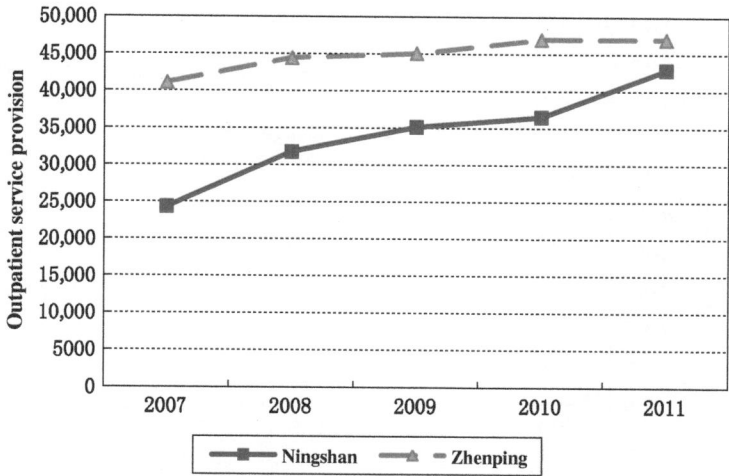

Figure 3.   The trend of outpatient service provision from 2007 to 2011 in Ningshan and Zhenping County hospitals. Data source: Annual operation reports from 2007 to 2011 in Ningshan and Zhenping County hospitals.

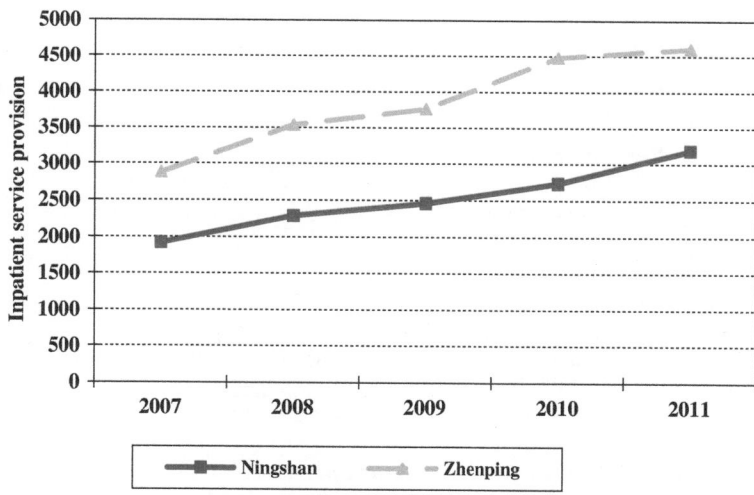

Figure 4.   The trend of inpatient service provision from 2007 to 2011 in Ningshan and Zhenping County hospitals. Data source: Annual operation reports from 2007 to 2011 in Ningshan and Zhenping County hospitals.

3.3.   The effects of zero-markup policy on medical service provision

Table 2 shows that the outpatient service provision increased in Ningshan County Hospital by 28.55%, from 33,967 visits to 43,666 visits between 2010 and 2011. The inpatient service provision increased by 16.17%, from 2729 visits to 3185 visits in Ningshan County Hospital. The outpatient service provision was similar between the year of 2010 and 2011 in Zhenping County Hospital, and the inpatient service provision only increased by 1.31%. Following the implementation of the zero-markup policy,

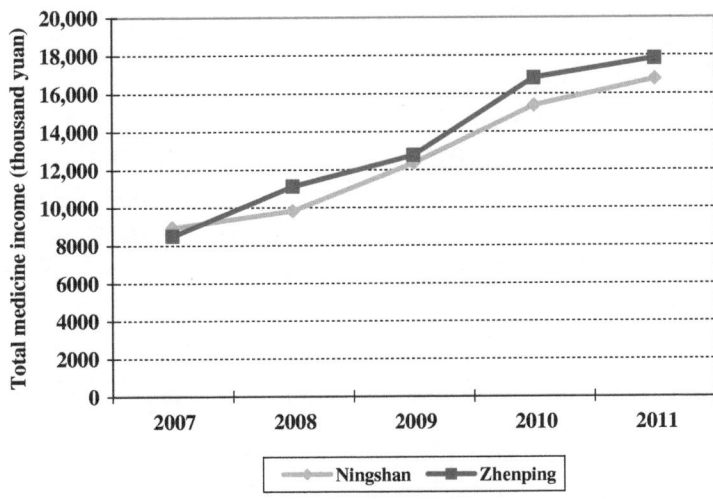

Figure 5. The trend of total health care revenue from 2007 to 2011 in Ningshan and Zhenping County hospitals. Data source: Annual financial statements from 2007 to 2011 in Ningshan and Zhenping County hospitals.

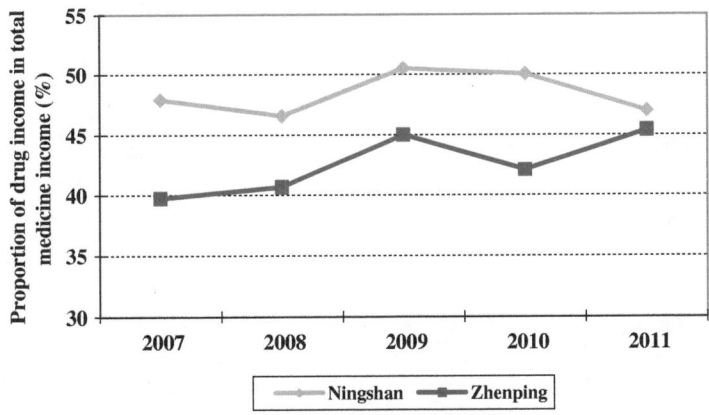

Figure 6. The trend of the proportion of drug revenue in total health care revenue from 2007 to 2011 in Ningshan and Zhenping County hospitals. Data source: Annual financial statements from 2007 to 2011 in Ningshan and Zhenping County hospitals.

Table 1. The effects of zero-markup policy on per-visit outpatient and inpatient expense.

	Per-visit outpatient expense (Yuan)		Per-visit inpatient expense (Yuan)	
	Ningshan	Zhenping	Ningshan	Zhenping
2010	168.00	130.25	3418.78	2394.03
2011	148.96	130.23	3182.81	2547.18
D1	−19.04	−0.02	−235.97	153.14
DID	−19.02		−389.11	

Note: D1 is the medical expense difference between the year of 2011 and 2010. Data source: Annual operation reports from 2010 to 2011 in Ningshan and Zhenping County hospitals.

Table 2.   The effects of zero-markup policy on outpatient and inpatient service provision.

	Outpatient service provision		Inpatient service provision	
	Ningshan	Zhenping	Ningshan	Zhenping
2010	33,967	46,955	2729	4416
2011	43,666	46,957	3185	4474
D1	9699	2	456	58
DID		9697		398

Note: D1 is the provision difference between the year of 2011 and 2010. Data source: Annual operation reports from 2010 to 2011 in Ningshan and Zhenping County hospitals.

outpatient and inpatient service provision in Ningshan County increased by 9697 visits and 398 visits, respectively.

3.4.   The effects of zero-markup policy on the health care revenue for hospitals

There are three sources of revenue for county public hospitals in China: first, medical revenue, which includes medical fees, examination fees, test fees, surgery fees, bed fees, and so on; second, drug revenue; and third, subsidies from the government. Health care revenue consists of medical revenue and drug revenue. It is analysed whether the zero-markup policy could change the total health care revenue, drug revenue, and the proportion of drug revenue in total health care revenue and total hospital revenue.

3.4.1.   Drug revenue in total health care revenue

Table 3 shows that Ningshan County Hospital's total health care revenue increased by 358.2 thousand Yuan, drug revenue reduced by 842.8 thousand Yuan, and the proportion of drug revenue out of total health care revenue reduced by 6.37%.

3.4.2.   Drug revenue in hospital's total revenue

The DID results in Table 4 show that, after the implementation of the zero-markup policy, the total hospital revenue increased by 901.2 thousand Yuan, the proportion of drug

Table 3.   The effects of zero-markup on total health care revenue, drug revenue, and the proportion of drug revenue in total health care revenue.

	Total health care revenue (thousand Yuan)		Drug revenue (thousand Yuan)		Proportion (%)	
	Ningshan	Zhenping	Ningshan	Zhenping	Ningshan	Zhenping
2010	15,374.8	16,812.3	7691.3	7073.0	50.03	42.07
2011	16,755.3	17,834.6	7874.7	8099.2	47.00	45.41
D1	1380.5	1022.3	183.4	1026.2	−3.03	3.34
DID		358.2		−842.8		−6.37

Note: D1 is the revenue difference between the year of 2011 and 2010. Data source: Annual financial statements from 2010 to 2011 in Ningshan and Zhenping County hospitals.

Table 4. The effects of the zero-markup policy on total hospital revenue and the proportion of drug revenue (subsidies) in total revenue.

	Total revenue (thousand Yuan)		The proportion of drug revenue (%)		The proportion of subsidies (%)	
	Ningshan	Zhenping	Ningshan	Zhenping	Ningshan	Zhenping
2010	19,928.5	20,093.8	38.59	35.20	22.20	14.68
2011	22,467.1	21,731.2	35.05	37.27	24.70	13.57
D1	2538.6	1637.4	−3.54	2.07	2.51	−1.11
DID	901.2		−5.61		3.62	

Note: D1 is the revenue difference between the year of 2011 and 2010. Data source: Annual financial statements from 2010 to 2011 in Ningshan and Zhenping County hospitals.

revenue in total revenue decreased by 5.61%, and the proportion of subsidies in total revenue increased by 3.62%.

3.5. Estimates of government subsidy

This study has the capacity to estimate the specific amount of government subsidy that was required to incentivize the hospital to implement the zero-markup policy. The subsidies from the government were 4420 thousand Yuan and 5550 thousand Yuan in 2010 and 2011, respectively, in Ningshan County Hospital, and the subsidies increased by 1130 thousand Yuan from 2010 to 2011. How much fiscal revenue should be allocated to implement the zero-markup policy? Two results are estimated based on two different methods.

First, based on the '15% markup principle', as the markup rate is 15% before the implementation of zero-markup policy, the government decided to compensate the hospital the lost 15% markup. In 2011, the total drug revenue was 7874.7 thousand Yuan (Table 3) and the proportion of the revenue from essential drugs in total drug revenue was 15.8% from hospital financial reports. Therefore, the government subsidy that should have been provided to the hospital is 186.7 thousand Yuan.

Government subsidy

= total drug revenue × proportion of revenue of zero-markup drug out of total drug revenue × the markup rate in drug sale

= 7874.7 × 0.158 × 0.15

= 186.7 thousand Yuan

This result is close to the hospital-reported loss due to the zero-markup policy in the year of 2011, which was 194 thousand Yuan.

Second, based on the 'natural growth principle', after the implementation of the zero-markup policy, the hospital health care revenue increased from 15,374.8 thousand Yuan to 16,755.3 thousand Yuan, by 1380.3 thousand Yuan and by 8.98% from 2010 to 2011 in Ningshan County Hospital (Table 3). As the drug price declined, the per-visit outpatient expense and per-visit inpatient expense decreased. However, the outpatient and inpatient provision increased, which increased the health care revenue. Even if the natural increase of 5% is considered, the medicine revenue still increased by 5%. Accordingly, the government does not have to provide extra subsidy to the hospital in terms of compensating any potential loss caused by the zero-markup policy.

4. Discussion

4.1. Assumption of DID

DID is based on the assumption that, without the intervention, the trends of outcome variables from treatment group and control group should be similar. In this study, that assumption is satisfied. For the outcome variables, including outpatient service provision, inpatient service provision, health care revenue, and the proportion of drug revenue in total health care revenue from 2007 to 2010, data were collected to reveal the trends of these variables between treatment hospital and control hospital. It is demonstrated that the trends between two hospitals are similar to each other for all outcome variables in the time period prior to policy implementation.

4.2. Correlation of per-visit medical expense and health care provision

Theoretically, after the implementation of the policy of the zero-markup in essential drugs, drug retail price will decline as a result of cancelling medicine markups, and therefore, the drug expense per outpatient visit and per inpatient visit, and the proportion of drug expense in total medical expense will be reduced. Furthermore, as drugs account for a higher proportion of total medical expense in the county hospitals than in other hospitals, the medical expenses per visit could be reduced substantially.

The results show that, with the implementation of zero-markup policy, the per-visit outpatient expense and per-visit inpatient expense decreased in Ningshan County Hospital in 2011. This is consistent with the results of Shen's study and Wang's study (Shen 2013, Wang et al. 2013), which show an overall decrease in health care expenses with the implementation of the zero-markup policy.

Meanwhile, the zero-markup policy made the outpatient provision and inpatient provision increase by 28.8% and 14.6%, respectively, in Ningshan County Hospital. This is consistent with the studies in community-level medical institutions (Chen et al. 2010, Tao et al. 2011), which show increases in health care provision with the implementation of zero-markup policy. Those results are linked to each other through the understanding of price elasticity of demand for health care. Data from China's National Health Service Survey show that both the price elasticity of outpatient provision and price elasticity of inpatient provision in rural areas are negative, which suggests that the demand for outpatient service and inpatient service increases with the decrease of health care price (Zhou et al. 2011). Evidence from this study echoes Zhou et al.'s study, which shows, using nationally representative data, that the price elasticity of demand for health care is negative.

4.3. Hospital's revenue

An important finding from this study is that for Ningshan County Hospital, the zero-markup policy led to a decrease in drug revenue. The proportion of drug revenue out of total health care revenue and the proportion of drug revenue out of total hospital revenue reduced by 6.37% and 5.61%, respectively. Despite this drop in drug revenue, the total health care revenue and total hospital revenue increased primarily due to the significant increase in outpatient and inpatient provision. This is consistent with the findings from a study conducted on primary medical institutions (Chen et al. 2010).

The zero-markup policy clearly impacted the level of drug revenue. However, as shown by Tables 3 and 4, the proportion of drug revenue in health care revenue and in total hospital revenue is still very high, at 47% and 35%, respectively. Efforts aimed at reducing the drug revenue to an even greater extent may include a variety of tactics, including changes in drug pricing, drug circulation, and rational drug use.

4.4. The government subsidy

Any effort to expand the zero-markup policy to other county hospitals will demand involvement by the government. As shown by the study, following the implementation of the zero-markup policy, the government's actual subsidy increased by 1130 thousand Yuan, according to the hospital financial records. However, according to the '15% markup principle', the subsidy-in-need from the government should have been 186.7 thousand Yuan. Based on the alternative analysis using the 'natural growth principle', we found that the government would not need to subsidize the hospital at all. This is because the health care revenue increased by 1576.6 thousand Yuan, which is a 5% increase.

If the '15% compensation principle' is applied, the government has to budget to subsidize the hospital, which is a suboptimum choice. If the 'natural growth principle' is applied for fiscal subsidy, no additional government subsidy is necessary. By implementing the zero-markup policy and the 'natural growth principle' for subsidy, more patients utilize health care at lower price and the hospitals have increased revenue, even without government subsidy, which is the Pareto improvement from the societal perspective.

4.5. Limitations

There are some important limitations in this study. First, the analysis of drug expenses was conducted with consideration of all drugs rather than specifically on zero-markup drugs. This was necessary because it is impossible to distinguish zero-markup drugs from other drugs in a patient data-set. Another limitation is the generalizability of the findings. Given that the study evaluates the zero-markup policy over only one year, it is difficult to generalize this impact into the future. It is possible that the policy impact only persists for a short period and then returns to previous trends. Furthermore, while the similarities between the two county hospitals in the study was a strength for this type of analysis, the external validity of the study could be enhanced by exploring more representative samples.

5. Conclusion

The implementation of a zero-markup policy in a county-level hospital is advancement for the hospital. For the county hospital, while the policy led to decreases in drug revenue, it led to an overall increase in the total hospital revenue during the year of implementation. This was mostly due to the increase in health care provision resulting from lower drug prices. The enhancement in outpatient and inpatient visits also represents progress from the lens of the government, whose mission is to ensure greater access to care for the population. The study shows that with minimal or no subsidy, the government can catalyse the zero-markup policy and potentially generate positive outcomes for county hospitals. Efforts to advance health reform should strongly consider the expansion of the zero-markup drug policy to other county hospitals in rural China.

Disclosure statement
No potential conflict of interest was reported by the authors.

Funding

This study was funded by the National Natural Science Fund of China [serial number 71203177]; Shaanxi Social Science Fund [serial number 12Q036]; and the China Medical Board (CMB). The funders had no role in study design, data collection and analysis, decision to publish, or preparation of the manuscript.

References

Center for Health Statistics and Information and MOH, 1994. *An analysis report of National Health Services Survey in China.* Beijing: Xiehe Medical University Press.

Center for Health Statistics and Information and MOH, 2009. *An analysis report of National Health Services Survey in China, 2008.* Beijing: Xiehe Medical University Press.

Chen, Q., *et al.*, 2010. Influence of the implementation of selling drug "without added profit" on the development of Beijing community health service institutions. *Chinese General Practice*, 13 (12A), 3842–3845.

Eggleston, K., 2012. Health care for 1.3 billion: China's remarkable work in progress. *The Milken Institute Review*, Second Quarter, 16–27.

Fang, Y., *et al.*, 2013. Access to affordable medicines after health reform: evidence from two cross-sectional surveys in Shaanxi province, western China. *The Lancet Global Health*, 1 (4), e227–e237. doi:10.1016/S2214-109X(13)70072-X

Gulliford, M., *et al.*, 2002. What does 'access to health care' mean? *Journal of Health Services Research & Policy*, 7 (3), 186–188. doi:10.1258/135581902760082517

He, P., Liu, B., and Sun, Q., 2011. Comparative analysis on the drug price of township health center before and after the essential medicines system reform: based on the sample survey of three counties in Anhui province. *Chinese Journal of Health Policy*, 4 (7), 11–16.

Hu, J., *et al.*, 2007. The study of economic burden of chronic non-communicable diseases in China. *China Journal of Prevention Control Chronic Non Communicable Disease*, 15, 189–193.

Jin, C., *et al.*, 2010. The study on zero profit drug supply and the corresponding reimbursement policy in medical institutions in Shanghai. *Chinese Journal of Health Policy*, 3 (10), 24–28.

Lang, Y. and Li, L., 2010. Investigation of compensation mechanism for drug zero profit in community health service organization in Yinchuan of Ningxia Hui autonomous region. *China Pharmacy*, 21 (36), 3374–3376.

Li, L., *et al.*, 2008. Evaluation and thoughts on the effects of implementing the policy "without added profit" to sale drug in community health service institutions of Beijing. *Chinese Health Economics*, 27 (4), 41–43.

Ministry of Health, 2010. *Chinese health statistics yearbook, 2010.* Beijing: Xiehe Medical University Press.

Ministry of Health, 2011. *Statistical bulletin of China's health service development of 2010.* Available from: www.moh.gov.cn [Accessed 29 April 2011].

National Bureau of Statistics of China, 2004. *China statistical yearbook 1987–2003.* Available from: http://www.stats.gov.cn/tjsj/ndsj/ [Accessed 1 January 2012].

OECD, 2013. *Health at a glance 2013: OECD indicators.* OECD Publishing. doi:10.1787/health_glance-2013-en

Shen, R., 2013. Impact of drug zero-mark up sale reform on drug use in public hospital. *Chinese Hospital*, 17 (1), 62–63.

Süssmuth-Dyckerhoff, C. and Wang, J., 2010. China's health care reforms. *Health International*, 12, 55–67.

Tao, C., *et al.*, 2011. Effect and suggestion of essential medicines system application on community health service institution. *Progress in Modern Biomedicine*, 11 (13), 2551–2554.

The State Council of China, 2009. *Implementation plan for the recent priorities of the health care system reform (2009-2011).* Beijing: The State Council of China.

Wang, J., Zhen, J., and Fan, W., 2013. Investigation and analysis of the effects of national essential drug system on medical expenses in different levels of medical Institutions. *China Pharmacy*, 23 (32), 2982–2984.

WHO, 2001. *How to develop and implement a national drug policy.* 2nd ed. Malta: World Health Organization.

Wooldridge, J., 2005. *Introductory econometrics: a modern approach*. Boston, MA: South-Western College Publishing.

Yang, L., *et al.*, 2012. The impact of the national essential medicines policy on prescribing behaviors in primary care facilities in Hubei province of China. *Health Policy and Planning*, 1–11. doi:10.1093/heapol/czs116

Yao, H., *et al.*, 2003. The evaluation of medical care income of hospital in different rank of Shanghai city. *Chinese Hospital Management*, 23 (5), 11–13.

Yip, W. and Hsiao, W.C., 2009. Non-evidence-based policy: how effective is China's new cooperative medical scheme in reducing medical impoverishment? *Social Science & Medicine*, 68 (2), 201–209. doi:10.1016/j.socscimed.2008.09.066

Zhou, Z., *et al.*, 2013. Assessing equity of health care utilization in rural China: results from nationally representative surveys from 1993 to 2008. *International Journal for Equity in Health*, 12, 34. doi:10.1186/1475-9276-12-34

Zhou, Z., *et al.*, 2011. New estimates of elasticity of demand for health care in rural China. *Health Policy*, 103(2–3), 255–265. doi:10.1016/j.healthpol.2011.09.005

Index